ANTENATAL GROUP SKILLS TRAINING

A MANUAL OF GUIDELINES

ANTENATAL GROUP SKILLS TRAINING

A MANUAL OF GUIDELINES

EDITED BY

Tricia Murphy-Black
Midwife, Research Officer, Parentcraft Education Project;
Nursing Research Unit, Department of Nursing Studies, University of Edinburgh

Ann Faulkner
Project Director, Parentcraft Education Project;
Senior Lecturer in Health Education, Department of Nursing Studies,
University of Edinburgh

with 30 contributors

An HM+M Nursing Publication

JOHN WILEY & SONS
Chichester · New York · Brisbane · Toronto · Singapore

British Library Cataloguing in Publication Data:

Antenatal group skills training: a manual
  of guidelines. — (An HM + M nursing
publication).
  1. Childbirth — Study and teaching
  I. Murphy-Black, Tricia II. Faulkner, Ann
  618.2′4   RG973

  ISBN 0 471 91138 0

Library of Congress Cataloging-in-Publication Data:

Antenatal group skills training.
  Bibliography: p.
  Includes index.
  1. Childbirth — Study and teaching. 2. Childbirth
teachers. I. Murphy-Black, Tricia.   II. Faulkner,
Ann.
RG973.A58   1988   618.2′4′07   87-10488
ISBN 0 471 91138 0 (pbk.)

Phototypeset by Dobbie Typesetting Service, Plymouth, Devon.
Printed and bound in Great Britain by Anchor Brendon Ltd, Tiptree, Essex.

Editors and Contributors

Editors

Tricia Murphy-Black   Research Officer, University of Edinburgh.
Ann Faulkner   Senior Lecturer, University of Edinburgh.

Contributors

Those who have contributed directly to the manual are:

Kit Bevan   Senior Health Education Officer, Gwent Health Authority.

Jean Bracken   Formerly Senior Midwife Teacher, Blackburn, Hyndburn and Ribble Valley Health Authority, now Director of Nursing Services, Midwifery and Gynaecology, Withington Maternity Hospital, Manchester.

Stella Brown   Health Education Officer, South Glamorgan Health Authority.

Edna Crabtree   Director of Midwifery Services, Blackburn, Hyndburn and Ribble Valley Health Authority.

Valerie Tickner   Director of Education, Royal College of Midwives.

Elizabeth Cruse   Health Education Officer, West Glamorgan Health Authority.

Anne Doyle   Former District Health Education Officer, Blackburn, Hyndburn and Ribble Valley Health Authority.

Sheila Drayton   Senior Midwife Teacher, East Glamorgan General Hospital.

Bob Goosey   District Health Education Officer, South Glamorgan Health Authority.

Joan Harris   Senior Health Education Officer, West Glamorgan Health Authority.

Dereck Hector	District Health Education Officer, Gwent Health Authority.
Vicki James	Senior Dietician, West Glamorgan Health Authority.
Helen Jenkins	Health Education Officer, South Glamorgan Health Authority.
Rosemary Jenkins	Formerly Senior Midwife Teacher, Mid Glamorgan Health Authority; now Director of Professional Affairs, Royal College of Midwives.
Margaret Johns	Health Visitor Tutor (Community) Mid Glamorgan Health Authority.
Elaine Jones	District Health Education Officer, Mid Glamorgan Health Authority.
Sue May	Midwifery Tutor, Mid Glamorgan Health Authority.
Beti Miller	Health Education Officer, South Glamorgan Health Authority.
Tina Owen	Department of Psychology, University College, Cardiff.
Elizabeth Perkins	Research and Development Officer, Nottingham.
Colin Rees	Research Officer, Combined Training Institute, University Hospital of Wales, South Glamorgan Health Authority.
Coleen Thomas	Health Education Officer, Mid Glamorgan Health Authority.
Anne Whatham	Community Dietitian, Gwent Health Authority.
Eileona Wilkinson	Senior Midwife Teacher, Blackburn, Hyndburn and Ribble Valley Health Authority.
Margaret Wilson	Nursing Officer, Community Midwifery, Blackburn, Hyndburn and Ribble Valley Health Authority.
Toni Williams	District Health Education Officer, West Glamorgan Health Authority.
Ena Williams	Health Education Officer, Mid Glamorgan Health Authority.

The members of the Steering Group were:

Tricia Murphy-Black	Research Officer, University of Edinburgh.
Jean Bracken	Formerly Senior Midwife Teacher, Blackburn, Hyndburn and Ribble Valley Health Authority, now Director of Nursing Services, Midwifery and Gynaecology, Withington Maternity Hospital, Manchester.
Edna Crabtree	Director of Midwifery Services, Blackburn, Hyndburn and Ribble Valley Health Authority.
Valerie Crowe (now Tickner)	Director of Education, Royal College of Midwives.
Anne Doyle	District Health Education Officer, Blackburn, Hyndburn and Ribble Valley Health Authority.
Ann Faulkner	Project Director, University of Manchester (until 1985).

Bob Goosey   District Health Education Officer, South Glamorgan Health Authority.

Elizabeth Perkins   Research and Development Officer, Nottingham.

Ann Thomson   Clinical Lecturer, University of Manchester.

Jane Randell   Health Education Council.

Eileona Wilkinson   Senior Midwife Teacher, Blackburn, Hyndburn and Ribble Valley Health Authority.

Margaret Wilson   Nursing Officer, Community Midwifery, Blackburn, Hyndburn and Ribble Valley Health Authority.

Mary Wilson   Director of Community Services, Blackburn, Hyndburn and Ribble Valley Health Authority.

Preface

This manual has been written as the result of an unusual research project—unusual in that the request for the monitoring and evaluation of courses for those who teach parentcraft came from those devising the courses rather than from researchers. The research was based in Manchester, funded by the Health Education Council and aided by a steering group with diverse expertise.

It is often stated that research has little effect on practice. In producing this manual, we are attempting to share research findings in a way that will be useful to anyone who may be involved in mounting courses for midwives and health visitors who themselves will be involved in teaching health education to the general public.

Broadly, we aim to provide a framework, with a variety of materials, for running a group skills course. We also aim to provide a checklist to help with planning and organising courses.

A brief history is given on the development of the research project, the courses, and the stages of evaluation and development within the two systems—the whole in the context of its application to antenatal education within differing health authorities. The purpose is to help health education officers, midwife and health visitor teachers and managers to put on a training course for midwives and health visitors. In the manual we have concentrated on groupwork and teaching skills, and given a variety of programmes, suggested sessions and exercises for inclusion in a course. There is little reference to the actual content of the antenatal classes as this can be provided either by the practitioners themselves, or if they need updating there are other means of providing for this, such as refresher courses. It is hoped that this manual will stimulate those who are concerned with antenatal education so that the teachers of the classes will be trained to respond to the changing needs of the mothers who come to them for help.

Ann Faulkner
Tricia Murphy-Black
Edinburgh 1987

Acknowledgements

We would like to acknowledge the support of the Health Education Council (HEC) who funded the project from which this manual arose. Particular help and support was generously given by Jane Randell of the HEC both during the project and in the compilation of the manual. Grateful thanks are extended to the members of the steering group and the contributors who were so willing to share their materials, and to the many others who contributed to the courses. Finally, may we thank all those course members who allowed us to monitor their progress, for without them the project would not have been possible.

Tricia Murphy-Black
Ann Faulkner

Contents

Definitions

WORKSHOP
A term used to denote that the course involves groupwork and that the attenders will be expected to be actively involved in the sessions, using their own experience and expertise.

COURSE
Course and workshop have the same meanings in this manual.

COURSE ORGANISER(S)
The person or group who make the major decisions about the course.

SESSION LEADER(S)
The person or team who leads the individual sessions—this may be any teacher from the Health Authority with the appropriate skills or there may be a recommendation that this leader comes from a particular occupational group.

COURSE MEMBERS
All those involved with the course for its duration—they will include the midwives and health visitors attending the course but may also include observers, teachers who will be leaders of other sessions, or members of Health Authority management.

COURSE PARTICIPANTS OR ATTENDERS
The health visitors and midwives who are attending the course.

Introducing this Manual

1

General Introduction and Uses

This manual forms part of the Family and Personal Health Programme of the Health Education Council. It has been designed in response to the need expressed by different health authorities to improve the training and development of those midwives and health visitors involved in antenatal education. At present there is little formal provision for such training within either the basic or postbasic education of midwives or health visitors. Although the emphasis in this manual is on antenatal education, there is much material here which may be useful for other groups within the nursing profession.

The manual provides programmes and suggested sessions for teaching, communication and groupwork skills which are suitable for informal education within groups. Checklists are provided to aid those who wish to set up such a course, as well as suggestions for the support of group leaders, and evaluation. In addition, there is a short historical background to the development of two courses. Resource lists for the course leaders, as well as background reading for those involved in antenatal education, complete the manual.

Chapters 4 to 8 have been arranged to group together those sessions which will help with the development of certain skills. Much of the material is based on the idea that groupwork skills are best acquired through the experience of learning them. Such experimental material has been explained fully, with detailed notes of group exercises and tasks. Other sessions which are more didactic provide some notes and ideas which course leaders/teachers might like to use, together with suggestions for overhead transparencies (OHT) which may be photocopied. No two teachers will approach or conduct a session alike—the teaching aids are just that—aids, to be used and adapted as the situation demands.

Chapter 7, *Group and Communication Skills in Practice*, could be adapted to situations other than antenatal education, with the 'Keeping up to date' sessions applied to the particular interests of the group. Although there is reference throughout to antenatal education, it should not be too difficult to adapt the material to the needs of other patient groups who the course attenders may be serving.

The course described here is intended mainly for health visitors and midwives who are involved in antenatal education and have some experience of running such classes. However, its content could also be incorporated into the training of midwives and health visitors, either as a 'block' within the training or as separate sessions over a longer period of time. Any nurses who are involved with groups of patients would be able to use these exercises and tasks and apply them to their own needs.

The Aims of the Manual

The aims of this manual are:
  (a) to provide those who are responsible for the preparation of health visitors and midwives (or other nursing group) with a framework and variety of materials for running a group skills course;
  (b) to provide a checklist which will help with planning and organisation for those putting on courses;
  (c) to provide a brief history of how these courses were developed, the stages of evaluation and development within the two systems, and the application of this approach to antenatal education within different health authorities.

Background to the Manual

In response to the concern voiced in the Court (1976) and Short (1980) reports the Health Education Council became actively involved in the training and development of the health professionals participating in antenatal education. There has also been a recognition both by managers and antenatal teachers within the Health Service of the need to reconsider antenatal education in the light of the needs and expectations of today's parents, who require a greater flexibility and involvement in preparation for parenthood. The value of involving participants in their learning has been recognised within health education, but many of the professionals have had little, if any, education for this form of teaching.

Recent research has raised questions on the teaching abilities of midwives and health visitors. Criticism of classes has included:
  —poor preparation of sessions;
  —conflicting advice being given;
  —lack of realism about the burdens of parenthood;
  —giving the wrong impression.
    (Perkins 1979a; Oakley 1981; Rees 1982)
Such criticism may be expected, given the evidence that the basic training of nurses has not given priority to the role of health educator nor yet to the development of teaching skills (Elkind 1980). There is also considerable evidence that communication skills, essential in teaching, are lacking, for example, Faulkner (1980), Macleod Clark (1982). Further, the situation is not improved at postbasic level (Smith 1979; Faulkner & Maguire 1984).

Midwives have little preparation for teaching (Brammer 1977) despite official approval for this role (CMB 1962; CMB 1980; DHSS 1976). Myles's (1985) suggestion that midwives' "expert knowledge of midwifery and vast experience in dealing with women during pregnancy and labour qualify them as unrivalled teachers of expectant mothers" would appear to be overoptimistic. The 18-month training of midwives, started in 1981, may bring improvements but it still leaves those who qualified before 1983 without adequate preparation for this part of their professional role.

Health visitors' training, in contrast to that of nurses, emphasises the health rather than the sickness model and includes guidance on health education, but here, too, research has shown that their communication skills are poor (Faulkner & Maguire 1986). Hyde (1982) suggests that health visitors without midwifery qualifications should not be expected to teach antenatal care, childbirth and early infant care, while a recent report showed that 25% of health visitors have no midwifery training (Robinson et al. 1983). This may account for Perkins's (1978a) findings which noted that health visitors lacked an understanding how to teach the physical preparation for childbirth or an awareness of current hospital practice. Perkins (1981a) also suggests that a major problem of parentcraft teaching is the didactic style frequently employed by teachers. Limitations included inadequate identification of the needs of the group, control of the topics taught, ineffective teaching methods, poor staff relationships and lack of flexibility. While management may contribute indirectly by prescribing a rigid syllabus and not allowing time for preparation by the teacher or continuity of contact with course participants, without adequate preparation of the teachers in communication and teaching skills, effective teaching is no more than a dream.

As long ago as 1979 Perkins & Morris defined three sets of abilities necessary for antenatal teaching:
   —understanding of human development;
   —teaching skills;
   —the ability to gather and keep a group together.

Although professional training may provide the first of these, up to now training for the last two has consisted of little more than 'sitting next to Nellie' or their own experience as learners, which will probably have been didactic. This latter may well lead to expectations of a teaching role which is authoritarian rather than facilitative and result in teaching initiated by the teacher (Flanders 1970). Within an adult group where there are mixed needs and abilities, involving emotional and life-changing events, initiation by the group members is required if their needs and expectations are to be met.

In 1974 the Leverhulme Health Education Project was begun in Nottingham. Its terms of reference were wide, namely "to explore the theory, practice and the teaching of health education in a university setting and to design a model system (of health education) for an Area Health Authority" (Anderson et al. 1980). Part of this research by Perkins (1975–80) was used as a basis for improving practice.

Collaboration with senior managers in two health districts where the need was appreciated eventually resulted in two courses — a basic course (Perkins & Craig 1981) and an intermediate course (Perkins 1982). This teaching formed part of the work of the Senior Research and Development Officer, with support from the Nottinghamshire Health Education Unit for these developments. After gaining experience in teaching these courses, and with the encouragement of the Health

Education Council, a handbook was produced for teachers. This was distributed on restricted circulation, prior to evaluation and dissemination.

The handbook was based on the idea that "good antenatal teaching involves staff being responsive to the needs of individual women and their partners" (Perkins & Craig 1981). It was designed to encourage the use of small groups, with the teachers providing a relaxed atmosphere which would make teaching and learning enjoyable for all. Discussion of new ideas which move away from syllabus examination systems, highlight student activity and provide feedback for tutors, would free the health visitors and midwives from the straightjacket of their own experience and increase their confidence (Perkins & Craig 1981).

Although the Health Education Council has been involved in antenatal education since its inception in 1968, the Antenatal Health Education Working Party was not set up until 1980. Its terms of reference were to explore:

> "the potential for health education in the antenatal period, with special reference to perinatal and neonatal mortality. Issues that emerged included the teaching of parentcraft in the antenatal period and the inservice training needs of the health professionals involved." (Health Education Council Annual Report, 1980–81)

This responded to the concern expressed in the Court report (1976) that guidance was needed on what information to give parents and how best to present it to them, and in the Short report (1980) which encouraged research into the methods of health education.

This present manual is a direct result of research which followed on from Perkins & Craig (1981). The initiative came from the Blackburn, Hyndburn and Ribble Valley Health Authorities and from Health Authorities in South Wales, who wanted to develop improved courses for antenatal teachers. The Health Education Council provided funding for these initiatives to be monitored and for the compilation of a handbook which would provide a means of sharing those ideas and strategies which were found to be useful within the experimental courses. Teachers were asked to contribute material which they felt had 'worked well' for them, for inclusion in the manual. The chapters which follow comprise that material for other teachers to try out and modify the ideas to suit their own style and needs.

Checklists for Action

2

This chapter is for those who will organise and set up the training course. Although some of the chapter stands on its own, some of the questions in the checklists cannot be answered until decisions about the course content have been made (reading Chapters 3-8 may help in making those decisions). There are three sections to this chapter:

—course content;
—setting up courses;
—course participants.

In each checklist, various aspects of the section are considered, questions raised, and suggestions made which arose as a result of the experience of the two groups who have been through this process. The checklists may be used both as an *aide memoire* during preparation and as the basis for a record of decisions made and the reasons for taking them at each stage of planning. If such courses are to take place on a regular basis the checklists may serve to show how courses develop. The two groups involved in the development of courses used different approaches, faced different problems and dealt with them in different ways. This is reflected in the checklists—the questions and suggestions have grown out of practical experience.

Course Content

What should it contain?

The needs of the midwives and health visitors (or other nursing group) should dictate the course content. The materials provided in Chapters 3-8 and the sample programmes in the Appendix may be useful in making decisions.

Content checklist

Aspects to consider can include:
* Previous training of staff;
* Local circumstances:
    For example, if there is only one obstetric physiotherapist in the
    Authority, it may be good use of her expertise to ask her to train the
    health visitors and midwives in the techniques of relaxation and
    exercises. This principle can also be applied to other nursing groups
    who need updating or refreshing in a particular topic as well as in the
    teaching, communication and groupwork skills.
* What will produce a good mix from the material provided for your staff.
* Can you provide speakers, and so on, for the different aspects — if one
    aspect has to be left out — will this distort the balance of the course?
* Would it be better to have someone trained specially so that you can put on
    a balanced course?
* What are the needs of your staff — do you need to ask them first? Are the
    staff unaware of their needs (i.e. quite happy with authoritarian teaching,
    with mothers who never ask any questions)?
* Do they need to have an increased awareness of the value of groupwork
    which tries to meet the mother's needs?

How many of the questions below need to be considered at this stage?

Speakers

Speaker checklist

* Who is available within the authority?
* Who, if any, need to be 'bought in' (consider overall costs)?
* Is there a good mix of skills and representatives of different professions?
* Do the speakers need preparation?
* Who will do the organisation?

MOTHERS/CLIENTS

* Do you want to use mothers (or other client/patient group)?
    — as a group to be taught?
    — to talk as individuals with groups of professionals?
* If so:
    — who will find them?
    — brief them?
    — organise and/or pay transport costs?
    — arrange child care, if needed?
    — debrief them, if needed?

Pre-course meeting checklist

* Decide whether or not to hold a pre-course meeting (assumes that attenders are nominated some time in advance).
* Where?
* When?
* Who will attend?
* Will it be used to:
    — discover the expectations of the attenders?
    — or tell/warn:
        — what to expect?
        — what not to expect? see Content checklist

Setting up Courses

Working group

Arranging a working group may be the first stage — before deciding on the course content. Alternatively, decisions about the course content may help in deciding who should be members of the working group. The nature of the course will involve those interested in improving the service to patients/clients by training their staff. The composition of the group will depend on local circumstances but could include the managers and teachers of midwives and health visitors (or other nurse managers or teachers) as well as health education officers where appropriate.

Working group checklist

* Do you want a group which is:
    — from a single health authority?
    — includes adjoining health authorities?
* Do you want a group which is predominantly:
    — nursing, midwifery and health visiting managers and teachers?
    — health education officers?
    — members of another appropriate group?
    — a mix of the above?
* Who will:
    — chair/co-ordinate the working group?
    — be the course leader(s) — those who make the decisions about
        content, timing etc?
    — be the main tutor(s)?
    — provide speakers?

Costs

Although the cost of running such a course may be provided out of the inservice training budget, the midwifery teaching department budget, or provided by the health education unit, decisions about who pays what, need to be made early in the planning stage. This is especially applicable if using the multiple-authority approach.

Costs checklist

* Who pays for:
    — venue?
    — catering?
    — speakers' fees?
    — travelling expenses of attenders (or possibly residents' fees if needed)?
    — preparation and distribution of programmes, pre-course information, and letters?
    — materials used within the course?

Venue

Venue checklist

* Will it be:
    — a hospital venue?
    — a community venue?
* Have you considered:
    — the travelling distance?
    — the effect of hospital venues on community staff and vice versa?
* Have you facilities for:
    — informal surroundings?
    — comfortable chairs?
    — space to move chairs?
    — space for groupwork?
    — privacy for groupwork?
    — audiovisual equipment?
    — relaxation and exercise equipment?
    — mats and pillows?
    — other equipment needed for a special group?
* Can the catering facilities cope with a sudden increase?
* Is it warm/cool enough?
* Is the ventilation adequate?
* Can refreshments be provided easily on arrival/during the day?
* Is there a library available?
* Are health education materials available?

Course Participants

Participants checklist

* How many?
    — does size depend on other resources such as venue, number of tutors
        etc?
* What mix of:
    — health visitors and midwives?
    — other nursing staff?
    — community and hospital staff?
* Do they have far to travel?
    — if so, make it residental? (consider implications of this);
    — can coffee be provided on arrival as well as midmorning?
* Are participants motivated?
* Have participants been on a teaching course recently?
* How much teaching training/experience have participants had?

Timing—Taking Staff 'Off the Job'

Timing/staff checklist

SINGLE HEALTH AUTHORITY

* Which approach — 5 consecutive days or one day a week for 5 weeks, or
    part of a block during training?
* Does this need liaison between organisers and managers?
* What will be the impact on service needs.
* Timing of the course in relation to staff and/or public holidays, peak demand
    periods, etc.
* How many can be spared at any one time? (co-ordination between
    managers and course organisers is essential).

MULTIPLE HEALTH AUTHORITY

* Who will co-ordinate appropriate dates?
* Are advance nominations required — if so how long in advance?
* Can you cope with last minute replacements?

BOTH APPROACHES

* Can attenders be only those who want/need to attend?
* Has their workload been considered on return to work?

In using these checklists, other considerations may come to mind which can be
incorporated to reflect local needs and priorities, while some parts may be deleted;
this process can lead to new checklists which are totally pertinent to the users.

Establishing the Group— Communication Skills

3

Once decisions on the course content have been made, each course will aim to provide a set of experiences for the participants which will lead to a model for their own teaching. These experiences can be designed to mirror those in which they, or mothers, may find themselves in the real world of antenatal education. Being part of a group is seen as a useful experience in itself.

This chapter gives details of four sessions, three using group tasks and one, a lecture, as follows:

— introduction to the course and each other;
— creating an environment;
— 'I never told them that';
— communications dos and don'ts.

Sessions 1, 2 and 4 concentrate on developing a group and learning how to communicate through group exercises. Session 3 is more didactic, the notes included here giving examples which are suitable for an antenatal education course: adaptation will be required for other groups.

Session 1: Introduction to the Course and Each Other

AIM AND OBJECTIVES
AIM That group cohesion will occur, which will enable learning to take place. **OBJECTIVES** 1 To develop sufficient trust between the individual course participants to enable free and honest communication to develop between them.

continued on next page

continued

2 To appreciate that the situation of participants in coming to the course and working in groups of unfamiliar people is akin to the experience of mothers (or other individuals) joining a group for the first time.
3 To begin to share the experience of groupwork teaching.

There are several components to this session:
  —introduction to each other;
  —making superficial contact;
  —empathy exercise;
  —the trust walk.

Introduction to each other

A general introduction and clarification of the domestic details is a necessary component of any course. Arrangements for refreshments, lunch, timing of sessions, and so on, need to be clarified and instructions may be needed on the formation of groups, whether there should be a list of group members or if the participants are to choose their own groups. Members may also need to be encouraged to join a group with some participants that they do not already know.

Following these formalities, each participant is given the opportunity to make contact with the other members of the course, including the teachers, so that all are able to share experiences. It is important that as many as possible of those who will be leading the sessions during the course participate in this introduction, since teachers, will be seen to be part of the group rather than removed from it. This can help to engender the notion of facilitation and joint learning.

Making superficial contact

This task should not take too long—about 15 minutes. Participants are asked to move the chairs to the side of the room after which the session leader asks them to move round the room and make contact with individuals using eye contact and some form of touch which is comfortable, such as a handshake or touch on the shoulder. Participants are then asked to exchange names only before moving on. If people tend to linger and talk, a gentle reminder that the point of this exercise is superficial contact should encourage them to move on again. After a few more minutes, the exercise is stopped and participants asked for feedback on:
  —their feelings;
  —the level at which they did or did not enjoy the exercise;
  —the ease with which they found they could make contact with so many unfamiliar people.

Empathy exercise

For the next section, the course members are asked to find a partner that they do not already know, and sit down together. The session leader asks them to talk to each other about themselves—their lives, careers, families, and so on—one person speaking while the other listens. The listener may comment neutrally, for example, 'I see', but may not give advice, interpret what the other person is saying or make observations drawn from her own experience. Each person talks for two minutes before exchanging roles with her partner—the leader of the session keeps time and calls out when the moment comes to change over. After this, each pair is asked to join with another pair and each person takes a turn at 'reporting back', giving some of the details she has learnt from her partner. This part of the exercise takes about 10 minutes, after which the group is re-formed and asked for feedback on whether:

—they found it easier to talk or listen?

—they remembered easily what the other person had told them?

This exercise can be repeated with a slight change of emphasis, by asking the course members to find another partner and to take it in turn to tell of a happy or sad event in their lives, using the same ground rules as before and each talking for about three minutes. In this situation, feedback is concentrated on whether:

—they found it easier to talk about a sad event or a happy one?

An explanation of these exercises to the group may help the members, as not everyone feels comfortable with them or finds them easy to carry out. The explanation could stress that the exercises are a means of getting to know a group of strangers and helping them to work together as a group. If they have found them disturbing, it may help to promote empathy for new members of a parentcraft group.

The trust walk

The object of the last exercise in this session is to express trustworthiness towards and to have trust in the other group members. This could form part of the initial explanation to participants to help them see the point of what they are doing. Each member is asked to find another partner and take on a 'blind' role by closing her eyes. Her partner guides her across the room, to a chair, helping her to avoid bumping into other people and reassuring her in whatever manner she feels is suitable. Roles are then exchanged, after which feedback is concentrated on:

—participants' preferences of role, i.e. leading or being led?

—strategies used when leading to make sure that partners feel safe;

—what made them feel safe when they were being led?

Summary of Session 1   The use of verbal and non-verbal communication can be emphasised as a means of promoting trust in people and gaining their confidence. Course members can be asked what parallels there are, if any, between their own situation in the group and that of women attending antenatal classes and clinics (or other groups).

Session 2: Creating an Environment

The specific objectives for each exercise are given below, although it has to be accepted that some people may not use objectives but prefer broad aims: they are given here as one possible framework for the session. Course members should be encouraged

---

AIMS

1 To demonstrate that a pleasant environment may be created by the way in which communication is encouraged to take place within a group.
2 To build upon the trust and co-operation established during the first session.

---

throughout the session to identify their own situation with that of women attending an antenatal group.

The following exercises are suggested:
— name game;
— how did you get here?
— non-verbal communication;
— backache exercise.

The name game

OBJECTIVES

1 To learn a technique which will help members of a group learn and remember each other's name.
2 To learn the names of group members and help others to learn names.

The course members are divided into groups of about 7 or 8 people who are asked to sit in a circle. In each small group one person begins by saying "I am (name)". The person on her left, says "I am (name) and this is (name)" giving the name of the person who has just introduced herself. This process is repeated until it reaches the first person again, who has to say all the names, indicating each person in turn. The process may be repeated by starting in a different part of the circle, and/or going in the opposite direction. When this has been done, the leader asks two people from one group to change places with two from another so that each group has two new members. These are introduced to the group and the naming process is repeated.

This exercise takes about 10–15 minutes and then the leader asks for feedback on:
— the way in which newcomers were welcomed;
— how they felt as newcomers;
— the way in which they helped each other to remember names?

How did you get here?

OBJECTIVES

1 To share experiences.
2 To explore the possibility of support for each other, for example, helping with travelling by giving lifts.
3 To explore feelings with each other.

Ten minutes are spent in asking the course members to share their experiences of getting to the course, what means of transport they used, was the venue easy to find, and so on. This may open up the possibility of giving each other support and help with travelling, and may lead to the exploration of feelings with each other.

This exercise usually provokes a great deal of conversation and relaxes tension. The point can be made that it is a useful activity with which to begin the first session of an antenatal group because it may enable mothers to arrange to give each other lifts and thereby get to know those who live near them. It may also be linked to their clinic visits, as these, too, may coincide.

Non-verbal communication

OBJECTIVES

1 To find methods of conveying feeling to another person without using words.
2 To try out these methods and explore the feelings evoked by receiving and giving non-verbal communications.

This exercise takes about 10 minutes. The participants are asked to find a partner and to discuss how they would express approval non-verbally, and then to try it out. They are then asked to discuss how they feel in response to this non-verbal communication, and how they feel when giving it. Course members are then asked to go through the same process again, but this time expressing consolation as, for example, in the face of bereavement. Actually trying to communicate in this way rather than merely talking about it is the important feature of this exercise, and feedback is concentrated on:
—what methods were used for expressing approval/consolation?
—what feelings did they have when giving/receiving approval/consolation?
—what problems were encountered when using non-verbal communication?

Backache exercise

OBJECTIVE

To demonstrate that strong feelings may be evoked by touching people.

The participants are asked to form pairs and practise on each other a technique for relieving backache which involves dragging two fingers slowly down each side of the spine; it will need to be demonstrated before they try it. After five minutes, ask for feedback on:
—how they felt about the sensation, was it pleasant/unpleasant and on what level;
—other reactions to the exercise.

The leader can bring the session to an end by asking groups of seven or eight to discuss between themselves the techniques they use to extend communication and create a pleasant atmosphere in a new antenatal group, and if they would consider using any of the exercises they have just carried out as a means of breaking the ice in their own groups.

Session 3: "I Never Told Them That"

AIM AND OBJECTIVES

AIM

To demonstrate some of the communication problems which may be experienced in antenatal education.

OBJECTIVES

1 To demonstrate potential difficulties in communication.
2 To demonstrate that group members may not always see the session in the same way as the teacher.

This session is designed as a lecture and does not involve groupwork; it can also be adapted to situations other than antenatal education. Some ideas which can be included are:
— an introduction to the aims of antenatal care, such as to prepare patients physically and emotionally for the birth of their child and his subsequent upbringing.
Although this involves all facets of maternity care, antenatal education has a role within this general aim. This session can include the following topics:
(a) What communication is—include definition, ask for members' views. Give examples of communication failure within maternity services (Boswell 1979; Cartwright 1979; Chamberlain 1975; MacIntyre 1982; Townsend & Davidson 1982). Give examples of communication failure—possibly from the session leader's own experience of antenatal classes.
(b) The difference between failure to understand and failure to remember.
(c) What is recall and how can it be enhanced?
(d) Our own misconceptions: for example,
— the needs of women in different social classes; for example, working-class women may not want to know;
— communication within the maternity services; for example, that both staff–staff and staff–patient communication is good.

Session 4: Communication Dos and Don'ts

AIM AND OBJECTIVE

AIM

To demonstrate practical experience of communication failure.

OBJECTIVE

To list the barriers to group communication, both verbal and non-verbal.

The following exercises may be used to demonstrate verbal and non-verbal communication barriers.

Non-verbal communication

SIT BACK-TO-BACK IN PAIRS

The course members are asked to give as much attention as possible to the person sitting behind them and for one of the pair to explain the signs of the onset of labour. Roles are then changed, after which feedback establishes:
—how it felt;
—how awkward it was;
—how difficulties were overcome;
—what was needed.

SIT SIDE-BY-SIDE, FACING FRONT

The partners are asked to sit facing the front, side-by-side and looking straight ahead. They are then asked to give their full attention to their partner, but without speaking. Feedback is asked for on:
—how it felt;
—the need (or otherwise) to talk.

The fact that this position can cause embarrassment and engender isolation—as sometimes happens on a bus or train—can be highlighted. The link can then be made with the idea that a group of mothers at a clinic like to see each other when they talk: thus, chairs arranged in a circle may be more effective in encouraging communication than if they are in straight rows.

SIT OPPOSITE EACH OTHER

Pairs of course members are asked to sit opposite each other and to give their full attention without speaking. Feedback will concentrate on:
—the embarrassment of staring at another person;
—the desire to look away from a stare.

This can be related to arrival within a new group and the common practice of inviting new members to "Come in and sit down". Other ideas can be suggested, such as "Come in and walk round" or the use of a display of visual aids to focus attention and act as an 'ice-breaker'.

COMFORTABLE POSTURE

The course members are asked to try whatever posture feels the most comfortable for them and then to give full attention to their partner. In this situation, an open posture is found to invite conversation, which is not forced or difficult.

Summary of Session 4   Some points from this exercise show that:
— attention is necessary for learning, therefore providing comfortable conditions with opportunities for both group and teacher to have contact will enhance sessions;
— introductions are made more easily if movement is possible;
— open, friendly postures will promote interaction more than words alone.

Verbal communication exercise

A recipe is chosen which has familiar ingredients and is of medium length. Four volunteers are required, three of whom are to wait outside the room. The leader reads the recipe clearly, without undue emphasis. She asks the volunteer in the room to repeat it to one of the three from outside who has been called in. The second person then repeats the recipe to the third volunteer, and the third to the fourth. The fourth person is asked to repeat the instructions which are then compared with the original recipe, which is read again. Each volunteer is asked in turn for feedback on:
—how he felt before, during and after the exercise;
—what he expected to happen;
—what he said.

Chapter Summary   This exercise demonstrates the need for a reliable source of information to be given confidently in a manner which does not confuse. It also demonstrates that the listener needs to know the purpose of the information as well as the key points, and may not remember everything. Information given which avoids assumptions being made and allows the recipient to ask questions will be more likely to be retained. This may be linked to giving information in antenatal classes or to taking a history at the clinic, and the need for careful documentation.

References

Boswell J (1979) Are classes 4 and 5 paying attention? *Nursing Mirror*, **148** (12), 24-25.
Brandes D, Philips H (1980) *Gamester's Handbook*. Hutchinson & Co, London.
Cartwright A (1979) *The Dignity of Labour*. Tavistock Publications, London.
Chamberlain G (1975) Antenatal education: the consumer's view. *Midwife, Health Visitor and Community Nurse*, **11** (9), 289-92.
MacIntyre S (1982) Communications between pregnant women and their medical and midwifery attendants. *Midwives Chronicle*, **95**, 387-395 (Nov).
Perkins E R (1980) *Education for Childbirth and Parenthood*. Croom Helm, London.
Townsend P, Davidson N (1982) *Inequalities in Health: The Black Report*. Pelican Books.
Williams M, Booth D (1983) *Antenatal Education—Guidelines for Teachers*. Churchill Livingstone, Edinburgh.

Teaching Groupwork Skills

4

Five sessions are described in this chapter:
— setting the scene;
— aims and objectives;
— teaching methods;
— teaching a skill;
— planning a session.

Each session consists of a short lecture, group exercises or tasks (either two short ones or a longer one), and a period of reporting back when all the participants can benefit from an exchange of ideas. Although these sessions can be spread out over a period of time, they are meant to be used to develop a theme and so are better grouped together over two days.

The sessions in this chapter have overall aims (see OHT 1) which can be used either to introduce the first session or to round off the end of the day (or the sessions) with a brief résumé of the content and the way in which the aims may have been achieved.

Setting the Scene

AIM AND OBJECTIVE
AIM To create an awareness of what constitutes the teaching environment. **OBJECTIVE** To identify aspects of this teaching environment which can be changed in order to facilitate learning.

Setting the Scene

AIMS

1 To give an understanding of, and practice in, the skills needed in planning and teaching a session for an antenatal (or other) group.
2 To enable the antenatal group leader to structure her involvement with the group so that they obtain the information and skills with which to prepare the mothers for events during the antenatal, delivery and postnatal periods.
3 To help the antenatal group leader to provide an environment in which learning can take place and which is also attractive to the mothers.
4 To acquaint the group leader with methods of planning which will help her to use the small amount of time available to its best advantage.
5 To facilitate a better understanding of the advantages and limitations of the methods of planning, teaching and evaluation.

OHT 1

This session is planned to make the distinction between those aspects of the environment which can be changed by the individual and those which cannot. The different room settings are explored and the influence they exert on the group is examined.

(a) How can the scene be set?
What will influence how mothers feel about the place where they come for their antenatal sessions? (OHTs 2, 3 and 4 *To See Ourselves as Others See Us . . .?*).

Participants should be encouraged to consider all aspects of the environment on which they can have an effect. Ideally, details such as the following should be elicited from the course members:

—general attitude of 'teacher';
—physical environment, e.g. curtains;
—type of chairs;
—introduction;
—hostess role (OHT 5);
—share first names, to facilitate later sharing of views;
—provision of a cup of tea;
—wearing uniform or not.

Those aspects which are determined by policy decisions at a higher level, such as the type of chairs provided, may need minimal discussion, emphasis being encouraged on aspects which the individual *can* influence. Discussion can be lively, with the leader summarising at the end on the OHT or a flipboard for future reference.

Group exercise

This exercise takes about 40 minutes and is designed to allow course members to examine the effect of different seating arrangements upon themselves. Seating is selected since it is the easiest aspect of the teaching environment to manipulate. Groups of no more than 7 or 8 are formed and a leader selected who is given a copy of the seating patterns (OHT 6) and instructions (see below). The groups are asked to try out these seating arrangements and the leaders to report back their group's findings. It may be necessary to emphasise that this is a practical exercise rather than a discussion of the plans. Feedback will focus on the reactions of each group to the different seating plans.

Instructions for group leaders: setting the scene

Look at the four diagrams (OHT6) and discuss:

1 How would you (the teachers) feel in each of the settings, (e.g. at ease, vulnerable, in command, etc) and say what the advantages/disadvantages of the setting are for the teachers.
2 How do you think attenders would feel in each seating plan (at ease, reminded of other settings, etc) and say what you feel are the advantages and disadvantages of these plans for the attenders.
3 Choose which layout you feel is the most appropriate for antenatal classes, and say why.

AIM

To appreciate the use of aims and objectives in group teaching.

OBJECTIVES

1 Define and differentiate between an aim and an objective.
2 Identify cognitive, affective and psychomotor objectives.
3 Recognise cognitive, affective and psychomotor objectives.

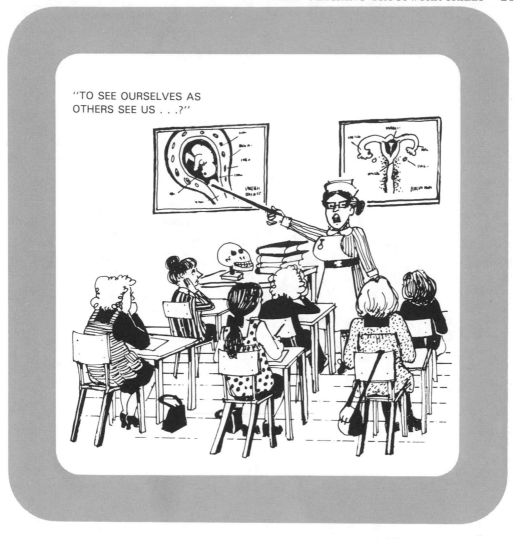

OHT 2

4 Formulate aims and objectives for a session.
5 Recognise the difference between teacher-centred and student-centred
  objectives.

An introduction often used for this session is the Sea Horse fable found in the preface
to Mager 1962, the moral of it being that if you are not sure where you are going
you might well end up somewhere else.

Defining aims and objectives

It is important to distinguish between the meanings of these two words.
AIMS—give the overall picture—think in broad general terms. They tend to
be vague and give a general statement of intent, for example, "To promote the

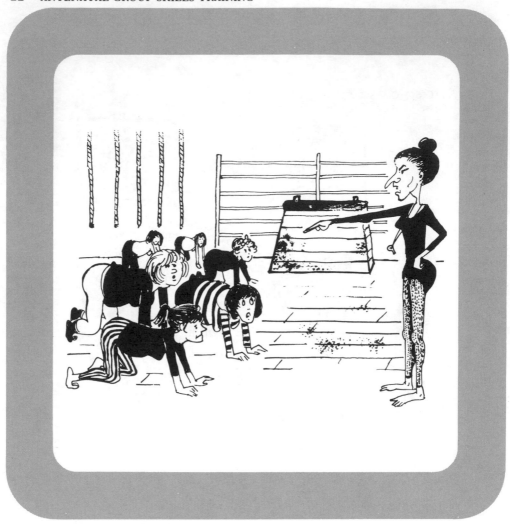

OHT 3

health and well-being of parents and babies". This sounds very worthy but does it help teachers to decide what teaching methods to employ.

OBJECTIVES—analyse the aims to arrive at specific learning outcomes. They are more specific statements of intent that describe a performance which demonstrates ability; for example, 'List five advantages of breast feeding'. Objectives should be measurable in behavioural terms.

Cognitive objectives relate to knowledge.
Affective objectives relate to attitudes.
Psychomotor objectives relate to learning skills.

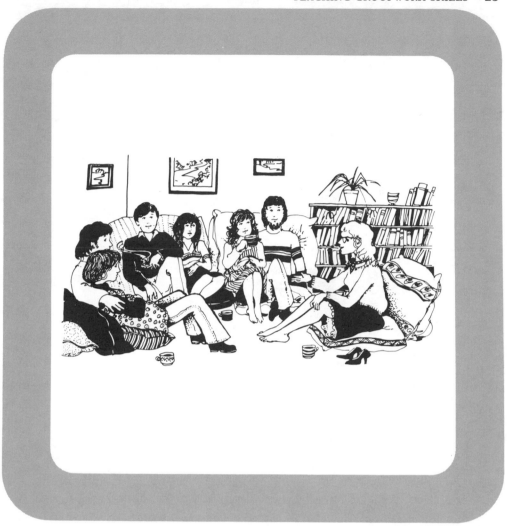

OHT 4

Importance of objectives

1 TO SELECT OR DESIGN INSTRUCTIONAL CONTENT

If people do not know where they are going, it is difficult to select a suitable means of getting there. For example, a cook selects the ingredients when she has decided what she is going to make, but the other side of the coin can also be true, that the cook decides what to make when she has seen what ingredients there are. The same may apply to teaching: the ideal is to have a clear idea of objectives but if the arrangements for a class break down (for example, if the film does not arrive) the teacher may have to be flexible, re-organise her objectives and teach with what she has available.

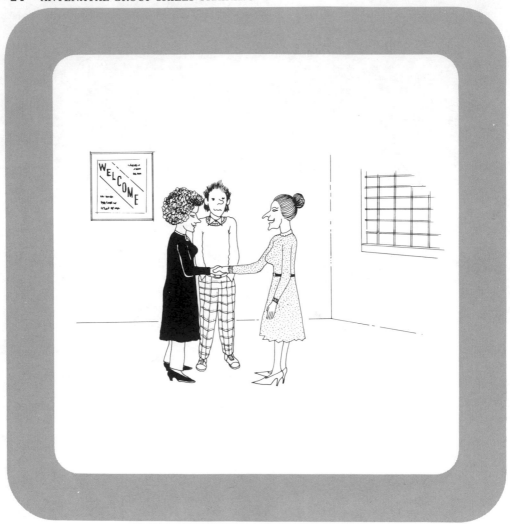

OHT 5

2 TO EVALUATE THE SUCCESS OF THE INSTRUCTION
(Have the objectives been accomplished—is the cake edible?)

An understanding of objectives can help to achieve:
  —improved communication with the teacher herself, parents-to-be, colleagues;
  —identification of the priorities in topics/subjects—even suggest possible paths
    through them;
  —ease decision-making about the appropriate medium for learning activities.

The instructional objectives place emphasis on what the 'learner' rather than the
'teacher' will do.

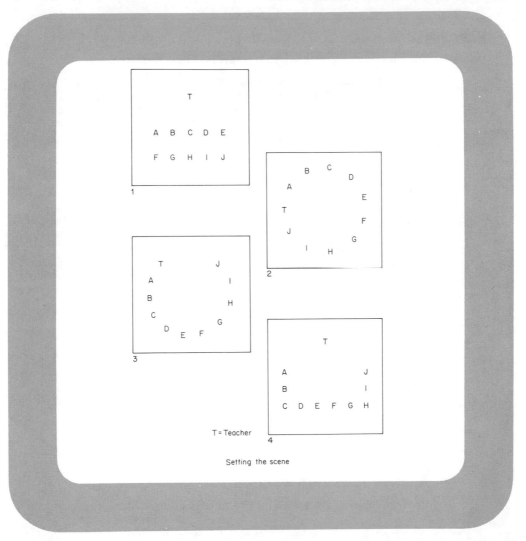

Setting the scene

OHT 6

Exercise 1

Which of the following statements looks like an objective?

1 Describe the role of the midwife and health visitor in relation to pregnancy so that the difference between their functions is clear.
2 Be aware of what midwives and health visitors do in relation to pregnancy.

It was said earlier that objectives are specific (so 1 above is more specific — 'describe' rather than 'be aware'). Care must be taken, therefore, when writing objectives, to use words that are open to the least number of interpretations.

Exercise 2

Underline the words which are open to the fewest interpretations:

> to know; to understand; to write; to appreciate; to recite; to identify; to sort; to grasp the significance of; to enjoy; to construct; to solve; to list; to believe; to compare and contrast; to have faith in.

EXERCISE 3

Tabulate the words to use and those to avoid when writing objectives:

WORDS TO USE	WORDS TO AVOID

(When the objective is stated as an activity rather than an outcome, you can convert it into an acceptable objective simply by asking the following question: 'What will the activity help the mother/father to do?'.)

OHT 7

It might help to think of objectives in three categories:

1 KNOWLEDGE—remembering and evaluating—thinking, concerns the information gained.

2 ATTITUDES—the analysis of feelings—self-growth, are concerned with values; for example, watching the HEC film 'Hello Baby' might produce a change of attitude towards play as an important means of learning. Change in attitudes is dependent on many factors: change will not occur if the required attitude is already held.

3 BEHAVIOUR or PERFORMANCE—the practice of physical activity—doing; using skills; relate these to the list of skills it is hoped that an expectant mother and father will acquire.

Exercise 4

The following objectives could be stated more clearly: reword them and tick the category(ies) — knowledge (K), attitudes (A) and behaviour (B) — that apply. In example no. 1, b is more precise than a.

	K	A	B
1a to be aware of the changes in growth during adolescence			
1b to list the changes in growth during adolescence	✔		
2 to know the methods of contraception			
3 to observe children at play and appreciate through this that a child develops both physically and emotionally.			
4 to acquire a basic knowledge of the skills of first-aid			

Exercise 5

Consider the four objectives given in Exercise 4; how would you evaluate whether they have satisfied their intent?

Group task

This exercise takes about 20 minutes and will need about 25–30 minutes for feedback.

It is planned to run a session for mothers early in the antenatal period, i.e. at 12–16 weeks.

DISCUSS
1 an overall aim for the session;
2 five objectives for the session to act as guidelines for the antental group teacher.

During your discussion, it will become obvious that certain objectives are more important than others. For this task, the order of priority is not important, only the writing of the objectives themselves.

HINTS
Aims are general statements.
Objectives begin 'The mother should be able to . . .'.

In feedback, the aims of each group can be written on a flipchart, or OHT, followed by the objectives. This can help to generate both discussion and the exchange of ideas.

Teaching Methods

AIMS AND OBJECTIVES

AIMS

By the end of this session, the course participants will have become aware of the variety of teaching methods which can be used at antenatal classes and, in particular, their advantages and disadvantages.

OBJECTIVES

1 List a variety of teaching methods, and their advantages and disadvantages for antenatal groups.
2 Identify appropriate teaching methods for achieving a stated objective.

This session consists of both a lecture and group exercises. The first part is a series of notes and OHTs which may help in presenting the different teaching methods. The second part, the group exercise, has an outline lesson plan which will have to be distributed to the course members.

Since the experience of group members, in terms of teaching experience, may vary considerably, some thought has to be given to presenting teaching methods so that interest is maintained. Using the experience within the group and sharing knowledge can allow all members to feel that they are involved.

Notes for lecture

The deliberate use of teaching 'gaffes' during the session to demonstrate particular points can bring some variety to it, especially if participants are asked to spot the mistakes! Among the possibilities are:
- showing a film at the silent speed—a common event—(the voice is slow and deep);
- standing between the overhead projector and the screen;
- forgetting to remove the masking paper on a transparency;
- speaking with head down, allowing no eye contact with the group;
- not speaking clearly;
- continually using unessential words or phrases; e.g. 'actually'; 'I am sure you are aware of'; etc;
- writing too small or illegibly on the flip board;
- using a marker on the flip board that is dried out;
- using a poor colour marker—pale yellow on white;
- turning one's back on the audience;
- using a flannelgraph where the pieces do not stick and keep falling off;
- demonstrating nappy changing having mislaid the pin or, worse, having no nappy and using a towel as a substitute;
- having a Betamax videotape and a VHS video machine;
- not knowing where the 13 amp points are, or, worse, having a 13 amp plug and 15 amp point.

Antenatal classes have the advantage in adult education that all who attend do so for the same reason—the coming event. They are also groups which include a mix of educational, social and cultural backgrounds. Participation by group members as well as listening to a teacher can both add variety and aid learning.

Teachers need to ask themselves questions to discover how much involvement and groupwork there is in the class:
- Is there a friendly and relaxed atmosphere which reduces anxiety and lowers tension?
- What type of leader is the teacher? This gives the opportunity to describe the three leader types:
  1 *authoritarian*—the leader who makes the decisions about what will go on in the group and generally directs the activities;
  2 *democratic*—the leader who involves the group members in the decision-making;
  3 *laissez-faire*—the leader who lets the group do what it wants without any active decision-making.
- Do they 'reward' the mothers by using phrases like 'Yes, that is interesting'?
- At the beginning of a class, do they outline objectives?
- Do they then decide which method(s) is (are) best suited to meet these objectives. Another fact which teachers need to appreciate is how little can be done in a class (this shapes the mind towards working out what best one can do and how to do it).

Teaching methods include

(the following could be used as overhead projector transparencies as a basis for discussion)

LECTURE

ADVANTAGES

    — all class members used to it
    — economical in time — covers more ground

DISADVANTAGES

    — no class participation — nothing asked of the student
    — proceeds at one pace — only suits a minority of the class
    — dependence on verbal memorising
    — no variety
    — no effect on attitudes
    — no feedback

OHT 8

DISCUSSION

More involvement of the members is expected and the teacher takes a place in it like everyone else.

ADVANTAGES

- — two-way flow of information
- — can identify gaps in understanding, knowledge, fears, etc
- — provides feedback
- — can modify attitudes/behaviour

DISADVANTAGES

- — some class members may dominate
- — shy members may not take part
- — needs careful control so that the discussion achieves its particular ends

OHT 9

DEMONSTRATION

Examples include:
- bathing a baby
- changing a nappy
- sterilisation of bottles

ADVANTAGES

Shows what a skilled performance should look like — this advantage is reinforced if individuals are invited to repeat the demonstration.

DISADVANTAGES

- unsuitable in a large group
- it is time-consuming if many actually do it
- timing may not be appropriate

OHT 10

AUDIOVISUAL RESOURCES

Aids can:
— invite co-operation
— attract and hold attention
— explain words
— illustrate relationships (size, etc)
— challenge
— consolidate

OHT 11

TYPES OF EQUIPMENT

CHALKBOARD, FLIPBOARD AND OVERHEAD PROJECTOR

— useful for recording key phrases and summarising
— diagrams etc can be prepared in advance
— with the OHT, the teacher can face the class and has more control
— also can be used in daylight

FELTBOARD

— useful for diagrams

MODELS

— 3D and life-size (people cannot always relate to a 2D diagram)

CASSETTE RECORDINGS

— allows participants to hear views of authoritative speakers
— can be edited if time is short

OHT 12

FILMS AND VIDEOTAPES

ADVANTAGES

- — can focus class attention
- — can influence attitudes
- — increases retention of learned material

DISADVANTAGES

- — associated with entertainment
- — lack of active class participation
- — loss of teacher control
  (these last two can be guarded against by careful planning)
- — may be too long
  (trigger films, to stimulate discussion, are designed to be short — for examples, see resource list)

FILM SLIDES

- — can be related precisely to an instructional objective

OHT 13

TEAM TEACHING

Are two heads better than one (for instance, midwife and health visitor sharing a session)?

ADVANTAGES

- — pooled specialist interests of members
- — members of a team learn from one another
- — team support

DISADVANTAGES

- — expensive in (wo)manpower terms
- — needs co-ordination
- — incompatibility of staff
- — can be dominated by one member

OHT 14

QUESTIONS TO ASK YOURSELF WHEN THE CLASS ENDS

Was the introduction effective in arousing interest?
Was the content adequate, given the time available?
Was the time adequately divided among the various parts of
   the lesson?
Was the interest maintained?
Were the teaching aids and their use adequate?

OHT 15

It is worth remembering that as this is the age of sophisticated aids an old Chinese proverb supports the need for resources:

I hear and I forget,
I see and I remember,
I do and I understand.

Hiring equipment and setting it up needs planning and can be time-consuming.

This part of the session could take about 30 minutes with the following 45 minutes spent on the group task (see below) and 30 for the report back.

Group task

Each group is asked to produce a lesson plan for a two-hour session (including 15 minutes for tea), the aim of the session being either:

the preparation of a father-to-be for his new role, after the birth;

or

the preparation of a father-to-be for his new role, before the birth.

Prepare a lesson plan on the sheet in the following way:
— list the objectives;
— allocate time;
— identify the teaching method used;
— list the appropriate teaching aids it was proposed to use.

LESSON PLAN

AIM . . . .

TIME	OBJECTIVE	METHOD	AID

Teaching a Skill

AIM AND OBJECTIVES

AIM
To appreciate the uses of teaching a skill and how to organise such a session.

OBJECTIVES
1 To list sessions in an antenatal course where teaching a skill is appropriate.
2 To list the advantages and disadvantages of skill teaching in the group situation.

GUIDELINES FOR TEACHING A SKILL

1 Give the learners the chance to practise whenever
  possible — this can either be in the classroom or at home.
2 Keep it simple — it is very easy to use unnecessary jargon
  (see below).
3 Keep it short.
4 Demonstrate and talk at the same time — this is not the
  same as the mothers will do at home.
5 Beware of diverting the attention of the group from what
  is being taught. This can be done quite unintentionally, for
  example, by wearing something unusual, thus: 'I don't
  know what she was doing but she has a nice emerald
  ring!'.
6 Ensure that everyone can see the teacher and the
  demonstration.

OHT 16

The first part of this session comprises a lecture of about 20 minutes' duration, followed by a group task which will need about 20 minutes for the exercise, and a further 20 minutes for feedback. Two group tasks are given, only one of which is used unless plenty of time is available.

Lecture

The stage has now been reached where aims and objectives have been set, the teaching method for the session has been decided and the room is welcoming. When teaching a skill it is very important that suitable methods are used to convey the message. There are certain guidelines to follow when teaching a practical skill to a group.

Very often trying to teach a skill is made more difficult by giving it more mystery than it deserves—be simple and be positive. The following descriptions— one simple, the other complex—of how to make a cup of tea will demonstrate the point about keeping instructions simple. Decide which version to read first.

MAKING A CUP OF TEA

Put one teaspoon of tea per person in a teapot, add boiling water, leave for three minutes, pour tea into a cup, add milk and sugar to taste. (27 words)

First, collect together the equipment required to perform the task. As this exercise is often performed at a time of great stress, it is imperative that the items should be available to all family members at all times. There are certain standard prerequisites for those items which may vary in the qualitative sense with aesthetic taste and availability. The bare essentials must be a receptacle which is constructed with the basic human anatomy in mind.

To many individuals the material of its construction is important, whilst to others it may be purely a matter of colour and shape. Into this receptacle is placed a critical portion of dehydrated organic material, rapidly followed by a measured amount of a solution of hydrogen and oxygen in the ratio of 2:1 which has been energised to a temperature at which vapourisation of the solution begins (note well: this is critical).

This receptacle should now be placed to one side whilst a further smaller vessel is prepared. The choice of this second vessel again depends on the chooser as to colour, shape, etc. A major choice factor again is its relationship to the structure of the human head.

A small quantity of the solution of organic material should now be poured into this second vessel. At this point there is much controversy about the use of various additives including other organic or synthetic compounds—again this must be at the discretion of the consumer. These factors aside, the solution can be qualitatively tested using a simple biological test. If this gives a positive response, then the solution can be assumed safe and be used to satisfy the mental and physical needs of the individual. (281 words)

Group task

The group is asked to devise a strategy for demonstrating a particular skill, perhaps chosen from among the following examples, and when complete, to try it out. The group will be asked to 'perform' during feedback.

EXAMPLES

doing up a necktie	putting on lipstck
writing a cheque	casting on knitting
using the telephone	opening a door
filling a fountain pen	making tea
sharpening a pencil	opening a matchbox

or specific to parentcraft,
    making-up a bottle feed
    changing a nappy

In feedback, each group is asked to demonstrate its 'skill' to the rest of the course members, who should all be encouraged to comment constructively on technique, teaching aids and so on. Some of the group may object to this exercise on the ground that it has nothing to do with antenatal teaching, in which case it can be pointed out that its purpose is to improve teaching skills rather than knowledge of the topics taught in the antenatal context.

Alternative group task

MAKING A VICTORIA SPONGE CAKE

Ask the groups to imagine that they are running a cookery class. The aim is to teach some women how to make a Victoria sponge cake.

Distribute a blank copy of the story board to each group and ask them to assume that they have all the utensils and ingredients they need. Ask the groups to draw in the frames of the story board a sequence of rough sketches showing the stages of making the sponge cake. For instance (1) assemble ingredients; (2) light cooker; (3) measure out ingredients; (see OHT 17). Under each 'scene' write the student objectives for each stage and state what category each objective falls into, i.e. attitude, skills, knowledge.

Planning a Session

AIM AND OBJECTIVES

AIM
To provide practice in planning an antenatal teaching session.

OBJECTIVES
1 To list objectives, key points to be covered and teaching methods to be used for an antenatal session on a specific topic.
2 To enable participants to gain the confidence to teach adequately in areas outside their immediate expertise, given adequate preparation.
3 To update knowledge of the effect that a particular aspect of good health can have on pregnancy.

As one of the objectives of the session is to teach participants that they are capable of teaching in an area for which they may consider that an expert is necessary, any area of particular expertise may be used. The field chosen will depend upon the needs and/or requests of local professionals but the principles outlined here can be applied to any specialty. For the courses organised in South Wales the services of a dietitian were obtained for this session. At the beginning of the course the attenders were each given a number of booklets on nutrition and warned that they would be expected to make use of the information contained in them during this session.

Lecture

This lecture, the first part of the session, takes about 20 minutes and is in large measure a revision of work already done during the course and a recapitulation of the reasons why the course is being held.

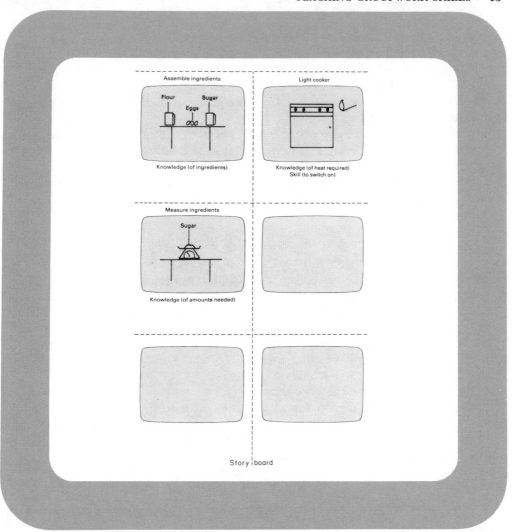

OHT 17

LECTURE SYNOPSIS

1 The teaching skill course has examined what is done in antenatal classes:
   —what is achieved;
   —what should be achieved;
   —what teaching methods should be used.
   The aim is to encourage questions from the group of mothers or clients/patients and to involve attenders.

2 To achieve the above requires the planning of both the courses and the sessions. A written plan is best because if information is held only in the head the teacher can be side-tracked.

3 In order to make a good plan the aims and objectives must be decided upon, and written down.

4 The structure of the session must be outlined:
   —how it will be introduced;
   —what points will be made in the body of the session;
   —what the conclusion will be—what is the punchline.

5 The teaching methods used to get each point across must be identified.

6 Key points summarised on prompt cards
   Prompt cards are index cards (5 in × 3 in or 6 in × 4 in) which contain enough space for useful information but unlike lecture notes, encourage brevity and can easily be updated. Key points are a logical series of points to be covered. Prompt cards can have other uses:
      —for questions to stimulate discussion;
      —to emphasise the important points;
      —as memory joggers for what comes next in the session;
      —to check that all the points for the session have been included.

Prompt cards are better than a verbatim script, which can be distracting, difficult to follow and lead to a dull presentation.

Group task

Taking nutrition or diet (or any other appropriate topic) as an example, and spending about 30 minutes on it, plan a session giving:
   — aim;
   — objectives;
   — key points;
   — questions;
   — teaching methods.
Each group should plan their session for a different stage of pregnancy:
   — preconception;
   — 14 weeks;
   — 28 weeks;
   — last class before birth;
   — postnatal class;

About 40 minutes needs to be set aside for feedback. The group leaders are each asked to present their session plan to the whole group. Giving the groups an OHT to prepare for their plan at the start of the task can aid feedback, and discussion of the plans presented. The session leader may make appropriate comment as long as it is not destructive, and encourage the rest of the group to offer constructive feedback, for example,

—on the objectives;

—on the chosen teaching methods.

Feedback also offers an opportunity to make a clear distinction between teaching methods and visual aids for the methods chosen.

Summary   In this chapter the sessions described have concentrated on teaching methods. Once the attenders have mastered these skills, they will be free to concentrate on the group activities. These sessions can also be useful for those involved in teaching in other situations.

Further Reading

Anderson D C (ed) (1979) *Health Education in Practice*. Croom Helm, London.

Davies I K (1973) *The Organisation of Training*. McGraw Hill, Maidenhead.

Ewles L, Simnett I (1985) *Promoting Health: A Practical Guide to Health Education*. John Wiley & Sons, Chichester.

Health Education Council (1985) *Major Programme for 1984-85*. Health Education Council, London.

Mager R F (1962) *Preparing Instructional Objectives*. Pitman Learning Inc, California.

Open University: 1 *Leading a Group* (£4.50; a booklet, part of the Community Education Package) 2 *Family Life Styles* (study pack—£10.00). (Both available from: Learning Material Services Office (LMSO); Open University, PO Box 188, Walton Hall, Milton Keynes MK7 6DH.)

Rodmell S, Smart (1982) *Pregnant at Work: The Experience of Women*. Open University/Kensington, Chelsea and Westminster Area Health Authority, 304 Westbourne Grove, London W1.

Rogers J (1971) *Adults Learning*. Penguin Books, Middlesex.

Runswick H, Davis C C (1976) *Health Education: Practical Teaching Techniques*. HM+M Publishers, Aylesbury.

Satow A, Evans M (1983) *Working with Groups*. Joint HEC/TACADE Publication (available from TACADE, 2 Mount Street, Manchester M2 5NG).

Strehlow, M S (1983) *Education for Health*. Harper & Row, London.

Sutherland I (1979) *Health Education: Perspectives and Choices*. Allen & Unwin, London.

Tones B K (1978) *Effectiveness and Efficiency in Health Education: A Review of Theory and Practice*. Scottish Health Education Group Occasional Paper.

Using Groups Effectively— Appropriate Skills

5

This chapter gives details of three sessions:
- —how groups work;
- —triggers for discussion;
- —asking questions.

The overall aim of the sessions is to give course members confidence, together with some insight into why and how groups may facilitate learning and attitude change. They also provide participants with some skills to use when working with groups. For two of the sessions (1 and 3), both of which have lecture notes and group tasks, the material included has been published and is not reproduced in full here. The middle session has notes for a lecture and examples of triggers which could be used by the course attenders in their classes.

How Groups Work

AIM AND OBJECTIVES

AIM

To give the course participants background knowledge of the formation and function of groups in general and when applied to antenatal education.

OBJECTIVES

"1 To give participants information about one or two models of group life.
 2 To help participants to relate these models to their experiences in groups.
 3 Through the above, to enable participants to recognise the value of having a
    workable framework to assist them in understanding the group they are

continued on next page

continued

leading, and recognising that if a group worker has appropriate tools for analysis she will be in a much stronger position to develop effective leadership skills.

4 To establish the fact that when groups appear to go wrong, it is not necessarily the leader's fault, but part of the natural processes of how groups operate."

(Satow & Evans 1983, p. 18)

Much of the material for this session can be gained from the HEC/TACADE publication *Working with Groups* by Satow & Evans (1983). Especially useful in this section are pages 16–19 on 'Group life', consisting of two pages of theoretical background followed by two pages of suggestions for using the material in conjunction with their videotape. This material can be used as it is or adapted by the course leaders for their particular situation.

Group task

The groups are asked to plan a session using an example of the triggers and to present this to the whole group; for example: what discussion triggers can be used from what is available in the clinic, when a film fails to arrive or breaks down.

In feedback, the group present their plans for the class, illustrating them, if possible, with the triggers which are available.

Examples of Specific Triggers

Statements/triggers

A list of statements and questions such as that shown here can be used in an antenatal class by giving a copy to each mother and asking her to tick those statements or questions that apply to her. The subsequent discussion can then be based on the lists that contains the most ticks, or, possibly, on those that contain no ticks at all.

Feelings about childbirth

1 I feel so unprepared—I just won't be able to manage.
2 I'm so nervous—it's the first big thing to happen to me which I haven't learned about beforehand.
3 I'm scared stiff—I had such a bad experience last time.
4 I'm frightened of hospital and hospital procedure.
5 I'm frightened of the actual birth—how can a baby get through such a small opening?
6 I worry about something being wrong with the baby.
7 Will I be able to cope with the pain during labour?

8 Why do I feel so anxious about it all—other women seem to cope?
9 I want to be in control of my feelings and reactions during labour.
10 I want to work with my body during labour.
11 I want to keep my figure.
12 I get very tense and anxious and feel I need to relax.
13 I would like to get to know how other pregnant women feel about it all.
14 I need to talk about how I feel to others who understand what its like to be pregnant.
15 I worry so much about little things—I suppose it's normal.
16 I haven't any maternal instincts and I'll never make a mother.
17 I want to breast feed my baby but I don't know much about it.
18 I worry about how to look after the baby.

Diary

A personal diary given to mothers at one of their antenatal classes and in which they can record their feelings as their pregnancy progresses, can provide a starting point for class discussion and a basis for mothers to use when formulating questions to ask in class or at the clinic.

DATE OF ENTRY	DATE OF CLINIC VISIT	DATE OF CLASS	HOW DO YOU FEEL?

Triggers for Discussion

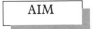

AIM

To stimulate the use of a variety of discussion triggers.

OBJECTIVES

1 To list a variety of ways in which discussion may be triggered.
2 To show, in discussion, an understanding of the ways in which trigger films may be used.
3 To list a variety of audiovisual and other aids which may be used to trigger discussion.

This session consists of a demonstration and discussion of various triggers which can be used to stimulate discussion. These will include (OHT 18):

EXAMPLES OF TRIGGERS

slides
posters
flip chart with key questions
a discussion of old wives' tales about pregnancy
a particular object; e.g. a feeding bottle, trigger
films (see resource list)
cartoons,
feelings about childbirth (see pp. 47–48)
leaflets
a diary (see p. 48)

OHT 18

Asking Questions

AIMS AND OBJECTIVES

AIMS

This session outlines the functions that questions can serve — and will assist in the identification of the difference between 'good' questions and 'poor' questions.

OBJECTIVES

1 To enable teachers to get greater participation from the group members.
2 To list means of obtaining feedback from the group members.
3 To demonstrate means of identifying the information needs of the group members.

Material for this session has been published (Rees, 1984), together with a group task and guidelines for post-session discussion.

Summary   This chapter has focused on the techniques needed for coping with groups. The chance to practise such techniques during the course can aid learning, although the participants may find it difficult to change from formal talks to group discussions, and may also need patience to develop their skills as they put the techniques into practice in their own classes.

References

Gillet J (1985) A helping hand. *Senior Nurse*, **2** (5), 15–18. A pull-out supplement listing support groups and organisations willing to provide pre and postnatal help and advice.

Kohner N (1984) *Pregnancy*. Health Education Council, London. A book with many pictures and diagrams about pregnancy, aimed at first time mothers. It deals with the emotional side of childbirth, together with the physical aspects.

Rees C (1984) Asking questions. In: *Education and the Midwife, Conference Report*. Association of Radical Midwives, London. (Available from Association of Radical Midwives, c/o 8A, The Drive, Wimbledon, London SW20.)

Satow A, Evans M (1983) *Working With Groups*. Joint HEC/TACADE publication. (Available from TACADE, 2 Mount Street, Manchester M2 5NG.)

RESOURCES LIST. Graves Medical Audiovisual Library. *Catalogue of Tape and Slide Programmes*. (Available from Holly House, 220 New London Road, Chelmsford, Essex CM2 9BJ.)

Films, videos, and tape slide programmes are usually available from the local Health Education Unit or Department.

Health Education Council trigger films — a set of 5 films each lasting about 10 minutes which aim to promote discussion on pregnancy, labour, pre and postnatal care, etc.

Group and Communication Skills in Practice

6

The aim of this chapter is to examine the process of obtaining and using, giving and receiving information in the practical setting. The sessions described here are:
  —keeping up to date (i);
  —keeping up to date (ii);
  —relaxation and exercises;
  —the mother's view and the importance of feedback;
  —awkward people.
The first two sessions are related and orientated towards antenatal education, and will help the professionals involved in such education to obtain the knowledge they want and need for their classes. This part of the course is concerned with the acquisition of knowledge rather than how to use it, with emphasis in the remainder of the course on how to use information.

It is suggested that one of three options is chosen on the basis of the assessed needs of the members of each course:
  —how to update knowledge;
  —teaching relaxation and exercises;
  —topics which are relevant to other nursing groups.
This flexible approach may require a pre-course assessment of needs before the programme is finalised, or it may be possible to determine needs at the start of the course if teachers are familiar with the material for all options. As the relaxation and exercises described here require eight periods or classes, there may be implications about timing and amount of content for the rest of the course.

The fourth session involves learning about evaluation and feedback techniques in a practical situation with a group of postnatal mothers. By using different target groups, the principles could have much wider applications.

The session on dealing with awkward people relates back to the session on group skills and although the lecture notes given are general, these can be adapted for other situations.

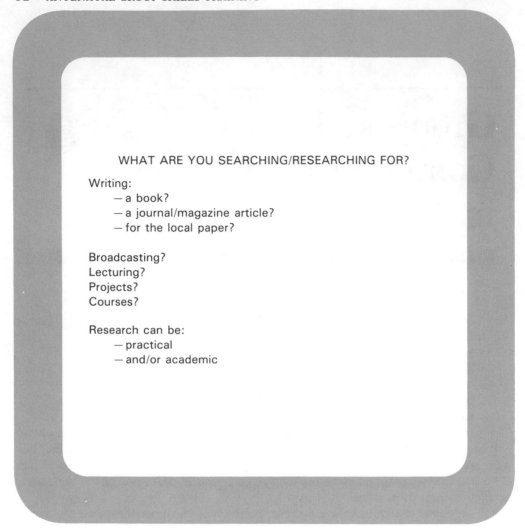

WHAT ARE YOU SEARCHING/RESEARCHING FOR?

Writing:
— a book?
— a journal/magazine article?
— for the local paper?

Broadcasting?
Lecturing?
Projects?
Courses?

Research can be:
— practical
— and/or academic

OHT 19

Keeping Up To Date (i)

Keeping up to date (i) has two parts which can be fitted into a session of about 75 minutes: both are lectures.

A Are we professionals?

Part A poses the question 'Are we professionals, and, if so, how are we keeping abreast with current knowledge?'.

   This session requires the inclusion of topical issues which will change from course to course and may be seen as an opportunity for team teaching by up-to-date professionals. It is impossible to give precise suggestions for the lecture here because of the changing nature of the material.

PRACTICAL RESEARCH

1 go to the source
2 pick up the phone
3 write a letter
4 ask friends and colleagues
5 use local resources — i.e. Citizen's Advice Bureau, Health
   Education Unit, libraries, shops, Yellow Pages
6 build up your own library and filing system
7 journal clubs

OHT 20

B Resources and research

Part B deals with research and resources and could include the following ideas.
It is essential to know the best route to any special subject if time, which is generally
at a premium, is to be used profitably.

As searches can be made at many different levels, it is important to establish
the depth of knowledge required for a particular project. Writing a book
will require far more research than collecting a few facts for a short talk or a newspaper
article.

Do not overlook the resources that are often quite close at hand. A phone call or
a letter can answer simple queries and a visit to the local Citizen's Advice Bureau
or Health Education Unit can provide much information.

DEWEY DECIMAL CLASSIFICATION

000   General works
100   Philosophy
200   Religion
300   Social sciences
400   Languages
500   Science
600   Technology
(610–619)   MEDICINE
700   The Arts
800   Literature
900   Geography, Biography and History

OHT 21

Literary searches are sometimes more time-consuming but knowledge of libraries and librarians can speed up the process considerably. Visit the local public hospital or medical library, explain the problem and ask for help. A good researcher is something of a detective. Aim to learn the classification codes of the library so that searching can begin at the right shelf. Most libraries use the Dewey Decimal Classification and most medical books will be found between 610–619 in the Technology section. Make friends with the local librarians and pick their brains.

Try to get access to more learned libraries in colleges and universities. This may require some form of membership, and even then some libraries do not allow books to be borrowed. However, these libraries will give access to more specialised books and journals than elsewhere, and reading in the library will be possible.

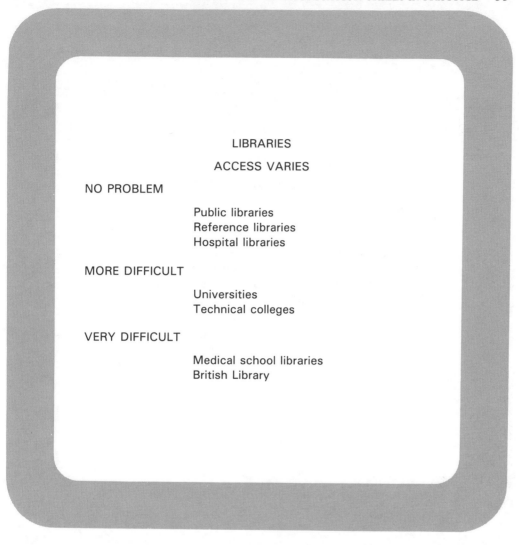

OHT 22

Some subjects can be daunting because of the sheer volume of the literature they encompass. One solution is a professional literature search, using indexes, or the help of the librarian who can arrange a computer search such as MEDLINE or NURSELINE. One problem with computer searches is that they can be expensive and may provide unwanted information. In both cases, the subject needs to be broken down into simple categories and titles, or 'key words' which precisely describe the areas to be searched.

Most indices work on a tree structure with titles, sub-titles and sub-sub-titles. Many of these are American-based and will have 'American' headings for their subjects. This calls for ingenuity—a typical example given by a librarian was a search on the topic of postnatal depression. Nothing could be found under this

ACADEMIC/SPECIALIST SEARCHES

LIBRARIES   LIBRARIANS

MANUAL SEARCHES   COMPUTER SEARCHES

— learn to use indexes   — ask librarian
— ask for: — have subject headings ready
  books and journals   — journal titles and abstracts
  through interlibrary loan

  Medical subject   Medline
  headings   science citations

OHT 23

heading but after an inspired guess all was revealed in the section called 'maternity blues'!

In all research work aim to build up an individual reference library. This can range from simple address books and filing systems to dictionaries, encyclopaedias, maps, timetables, and so on. Limit the researches only by the capacity of the bookshelves. Much time and energy can be saved if the information wanted is only an arm's length away.

SUBJECT SUB-TITLES

postnatal depression
postpartum depression
postpartum psychosis
puerperal psychosis
or
maternity blues

OHT 24

Keeping up to Date (ii)

Topic of current interest

AIMS

To choose a topic of current interest, relevant to the antenatal work of midwife and health visitor, which would illustrate how essential it is to keep up to date.

To show by example how midwives and health visitors (or other groups) can work together in a teaching situation.

Examples of appropriate topics:
— fetal alcohol syndrome;
— the effects of drugs in pregnancy;
— teenage pregnancy.

Detailed notes are not given here as these would quickly become out of date, but the lecture can include recent research, especially if it is controversial and has had wide media coverage. It should be something which will be relevant to the interests of those attending the course and about which they may be questioned by those attending their classes.

Teaching Relaxation and Exercises

The decision whether or not to include this subject in the course is dependent on the needs of local staff and the availability of a suitably qualified teacher such as an obstetric physiotherapist, a midwife or a health visitor, who has the relevant ability in relaxation and exercises, as well as in teaching skills. An appropriate plan is included here, but the final decision whether or not to use it has to be made by those involved.

Relaxation and Exercises

AIM

To enable health visitors and midwives to teach relaxation and exercises for use in the antenatal and postnatal periods, as well as during labour.

OBJECTIVES

1 To demonstrate the techniques of relaxation and exercises.
2 To provide an opportunity for the midwives and health visitors to perform the relaxation and exercises.
3 To provide an opportunity for each midwife and health visitor to practise teaching relaxation and exercises with her colleagues.

The sessions outlined require a total of eight hours to be spent on relaxation and exercises. Course members should be asked to wear track suits or other suitable clothing, while the session leader will need space for the exercises to be demonstrated and practised, as well as enough mats and pillows for everyone present.

INTRODUCTORY SESSION

General discussion on the meaning of relaxation:
- —the informality of the sessions;
- —catering for all social classes;
- —using simple terms;
- —promoting discussion and encouraging feedback even at the expense of the exercises;

PROGRAMME OF EXERCISES

A programme suitable for use in classes.
One or two exercises should be introduced at a time, and revised at intervals. Exercises for use during the antenatal period make a good starting point, combined with full relaxation and the opportunity for practice.

Throughout these sessions course members should be given the chance to practise teaching the exercises to each other, as well as actually carrying them out. This teaching practice helps participants to gain experience in using effective vocal tones and forms of communication.

The physiology of labour should be explained and talked through as the exercises are done, and positions at delivery can be demonstrated, together with pushing and panting.

Postnatal
Postnatal exercises may be demonstrated, stressing their importance, the reasons for them, and their frequency. The importance of correct posture, and wearing suitable shoes and clothing may also be given as relevant.

A Mother's View and the Importance of Feedback

AIMS AND OBJECTIVES

AIMS

To emphasise the importance of obtaining feedback about antenatal groups from mothers and to give some practice in obtaining it.

OBJECTIVES

To:
1 Describe what is meant by feedback.
2 List the reasons why feedback is important for both professionals and mothers.
3 Plan questions which, in an informal situation, will elicit feedback about antenatal groups.
4 Practise obtaining feedback in an informal situation.
5 List various situations in which feedback might be obtained.

continued on next page

---

continued

6 Describe ways in which teaching aids such as leaflets can be used to obtain feedback.

A mother's view

INTRODUCTION

In keeping with the philosophy that the experiential aspects of the course are much the most important, emphasis falls heavily on the aim of practising how to gain feedback from mothers. To fulfill this aim, some mothers in the area who have recently had babies are invited in for the afternoon. Although scheduled as two sessions, this afternoon can be run as an integrated whole. After a session on the value of feedback, the course participants divide into groups, and each group is allotted one of the mothers. Course members then are given the opportunity to practise obtaining feedback from 'real people'. This allows the idea of providing a supportive atmosphere for mothers in antenatal classes to be translated into practice, along with the listening skills touched on at the beginning of the course. The course leader will need to meet the mothers before the session to brief them about the session and to assess the need for child care or other support. The session is likely to be most successful if women from a variety of backgrounds and who have had different experiences of what the NHS can offer are present.

Because of the involvement of mothers, this session tends to be both enjoyable and worthwhile, but it can be unpredictable. Experience shows that the mothers always contribute willingly and do not seem to be put off by knowing that they are part of a training course programme. The session also appears to bring out the best in the professionals as they plan their approaches and questions. A typical afternoon goes as follows:

—a 15-minute introductory lecture;
—a group task (30 minutes);
—break for tea;
—groupwork with mothers for about 30 minutes;
—30 minutes in which to report back the groups' experiences to all the attenders.

Importance of feedback

DIDACTIC SESSION

An introduction, lasting about 15 minutes, to include some of the following ideas (OHT 25):

WHAT IS FEEDBACK?

Feedback is a two-way process.

In antenatal groups it gives both professionals and mothers the chance to find out if they are getting the most they can out of their group sessions.

OHT 25

Teachers are constantly giving feedback to mothers. What does this feedback achieve?

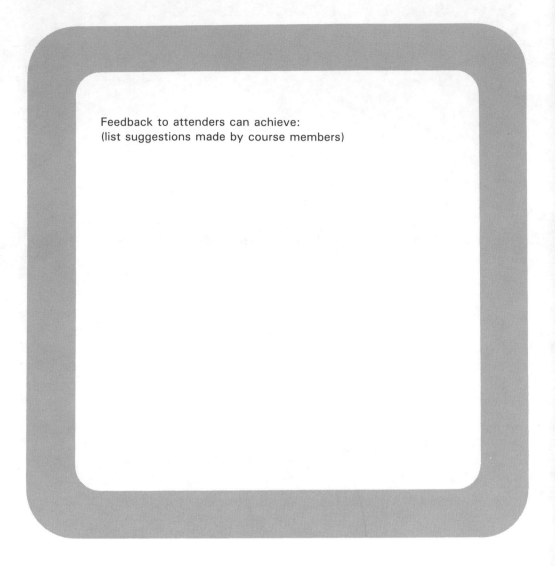

Feedback to attenders can achieve:
(list suggestions made by course members)

OHT 26

It is also important to seek feedback from attenders at antenatal groups as this can give valuable information on how the groups are going. This feedback, which is most useful in planning courses, does not always come automatically: when and how to obtain it needs preparation beforehand. Feedback is relevant to all aspects of antenatal groupwork: it can be obtained while a session is going on and will thus let the teacher know whether she is getting her points across. Feedback during a session can take the following forms (OHT 27):

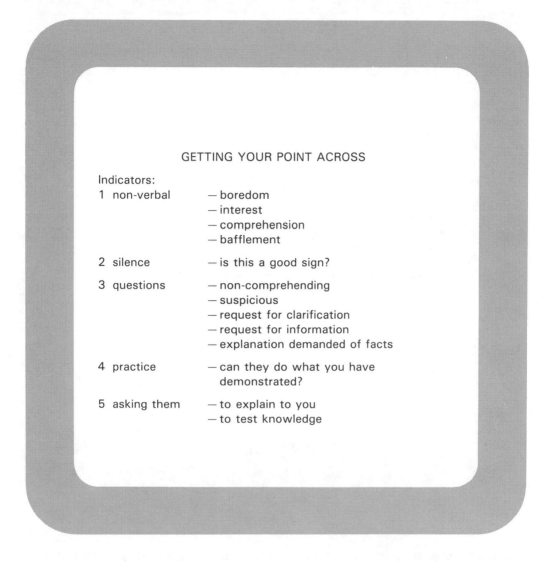

GETTING YOUR POINT ACROSS

Indicators:
1 non-verbal   — boredom
                 — interest
                 — comprehension
                 — bafflement

2 silence   — is this a good sign?

3 questions   — non-comprehending
                 — suspicious
                 — request for clarification
                 — request for information
                 — explanation demanded of facts

4 practice   — can they do what you have
                   demonstrated?

5 asking them   — to explain to you
                 — to test knowledge

OHT 27

Feedback may also be obtained after a session, and at the end of a course. It is the only way of finding out whether the classes are meeting the needs of the mothers.

EXAMPLES OF SITUATIONS IN WHICH FEEDBACK MAY BE OBTAINED

1 during and at the end of group discussions
2 during home visits
3 in the postnatal ward
4 talking to postnatal mothers
5 during a fathers' evening
6 asking questions of colleagues
7 when talking to newly-delivered mothers, either individually or in postnatal groups

OHT 28

Although these are informal situations, nevertheless it is important to plan how to use them to obtain feedback. This session provides the opportunity to practise one way of gaining useful feedback from mothers in a particular situation. Explain that mothers will be present at the following session and ask course members to concentrate on putting them at their ease and on finding out how they feel about the antenatal classes that they have attended.

Group task

The group are asked to plan a series of questions which will help them to obtain feedback from a recently delivered mother about one of the following:
- feeding;
- the preparation she received for labour;
- the relationship between a mother and her newborn baby;
- coping with a baby at home.

The aim of the exercise is to determine how well the antenatal group session on that subject has met the mother's needs and/or the midwife's or health visitor's objectives.

After this task is completed, and the tea break is over, the groups are reformed and introduced to the mothers to be interviewed. If the groups spend about 30 minutes with the mothers, 30 minutes will be left for a plenary session in which the leaders present the questions (on an OHT) which their groups used. The questions can be discussed in terms of their objectives and whether they were achieved. The course leader may also use this opportunity to recapitulate the principles of different types of question.

Other methods which can be used to obtain feedback may be discussed along with its value in antenatal teaching. It is possible in this part to discuss the pros and cons of handing out leaflets, and so on, and whether these aid understanding (for an example, see Perkins' book (1980b) from p. 67 onwards).

The use of leaflets for reinforcement of the point made during the class could be linked with feedback. If antenatal teachers discover that mothers have misunderstood certain points, or missed them altogether, it helps the teachers to consider both their own approach to the subject and to those aspects that require reinforcing. There is an old saying, much beloved of broadcasters and others, which goes:

"tell 'em what you're going to tell 'em;

tell 'em;

tell 'em what you've told 'em!"

which can be useful to remember in this situation.

Awkward People

AIM AND OBJECTIVES

AIM

To increase skill in dealing with difficult group members.

OBJECTIVES

1 To identify a range of difficult behaviours.
2 To produce a list of alternative coping strategies.
3 To provide an alternative way of looking at awkward people.

This session is mainly didactic with some short exercises for the whole group rather than small groups.

All participants are likely to have had the experience of being the leader or a member of a group where things would have gone much more smoothly but for the behaviour of one or two difficult members who are then labelled 'awkward people'. An analysis of what it is that 'awkward' group members do that is seen to be difficult is useful, and is therefore the subject of this session. Perhaps a good starting point is to think of ways in which someone might deliberately set out to be difficult or 'awkward' as a member of a group.

Exercise

Each person is asked to complete this sentence:

"I could sabotage the group by . . . ."

Feedback

The examples given can be grouped under a number of headings, for example:
   —non-verbal, physical;
   —personal attacks (verbal)/criticism;
   —ververbalisation/inappropriate verbalisation;
Since the problem is how to cope with difficult situations, group members' experiences of dealing with these kinds of problems can be shared to find examples of how they might be resolved.

Exercise

The course attenders are asked how they would cope with the following types of group member, which are familiar to all. It soon becomes clear that each situation needs a different approach.

The course members are asked to consider the following questions:
   —what may be responsible for the deviant behaviour? (is it possible to understand their personalities as a guide to their behaviour?)
   —what are possible ways of dealing with disruptive behaviour?

In feedback, the notion that there is no such thing as problem people, only people with problems, may be considered, and also why it is important to try to establish what lies behind behaviour which may cause problems in a group.

It is important first of all to identify the size of the problem, whose problem it is and its nature, before taking any action.

HOW TO COPE WITH

1 the CHATTY person who jumps in on each and every occasion with comments and anecdotes;
2 the person who DISAGREES with everything said;
3 the QUIET person who never says a word.

OHT 29

The size of the problem

Is the problem occasional or does it occur regularly?
Is the behaviour disruptive or simply irritating? For example, "Wouldn't it be nice if she didn't keep going on and on about her sister and her baby?".

Where the problem lies

It is useful to look on OHT 30 at the effect of the awkward person's behaviour.

EFFECTS OF AWKWARD BEHAVIOUR

1 THE GROUP LEADER

How do the leaders feel about it — how do they respond and behave?

Is there anything the group leader or anybody else does, that seems to cause or reinforce the behaviour of the person concerned — arguing with them, being defensive — allowing them to get away with being too chatty — would changes in the behaviour of the group leader help at all?

2 OTHER GROUP MEMBERS

Do they seem to experience difficulties as a result of the behaviour of the person in question — how do they feel or react — is it a problem for them?

3 THE GROUP TASKS

Does the awkward person's behaviour prevent the group achieving its task, or is the effect limited or even helpful (tension release), is it simply irritating rather than a major hindrance?

4 THE AWKWARD PERSON HERSELF

Is the person gaining or losing by the behaviour, what is the 'pay-off' for her? Some people will accept scorn or other people's anger because it brings them the attention they are seeking. If the pay-offs are recognised, then it might be possible to give the attention they are seeking in some other form, such as asking for their opinion and praising the positive rather than the negative responses.

OHT 30

How can the group leader change the situation?

1 Can they establish with the awkward person what she would like them to do differently?
2 Can the leaders offer help towards such a change and find reasons, in the person's own interests, that might make her willing to change? For example, saying to a talkative person "I think some of the others are letting you do all the talking—I wonder if you can help me bring them in a bit—if you wait for a minute or ask some of the others if they agree with you."

3 Can the leaders change their own behaviour in a way that could help that person—are they being very dogmatic—so that it is easy to disagree with the leaders—could the talk switch to talk of possibilities and options?
4 Can the group make any changes that would help the awkward ones—such as being more supportive or allow participation from the quiet/shy/withdrawn person.

It is sometimes helpful to consider, when labelling someone as 'awkward', that there will be occasions when others will regard the leader as being awkward. Some people seem to be more generally awkward than others but it is important to remember that everyone has the potential to be awkward and may sometimes actually be difficult towards others. Think back over the course: have there been occasions when any members seemed always to have something to say, chatting with neighbours, and so on? If leaders are aware of the factors that influence their own behaviour on those occasions, this awareness may help them to understand the behaviour of people who they find awkward.

It can also help to realise that other people's behaviour represents their reactions to their current situation. In a group this may be due to the behaviour of the leader or to group members' actions and behaviour. If the group leaders can gain insight by analysis of the effects of their behaviour, they may see the need to adapt their style in an attempt to modify a disruptive situation.

Awkward people have been considered here as being potentially destructive. Often those who interrupt the session or do not go along with the ideas or views of the group are seen in a negative way rather than as different people with a different viewpoint to offer.

Constructive use of awkward people

Working towards using the contributions of awkward people in a positive way may lead to more harmony in a group. If group leaders can remain cool about apparently irrelevant or critical comments, value may be found in them by which the contribution can be used in some way to relate back to the main theme or to move on to another area or topic.

People who disagree may actually be helpful—they may have come across something the group leader has not thought or heard of which they are prepared to share with the group.

Asking group members to be precise and specific about their question or criticism can be useful, especially if they can be persuaded to explain it a bit further or give an example. Comments which may appear critical or challenging initially may turn out to be genuine queries rather than criticisms, once they are discussed.

In order to respond to the needs of the group, leaders should have the confidence to be open to the contribution made by the attenders. This allows true group participation without an oversensitive reaction that everything is a personal attack.

It is worth remembering that negative feedback seldom changes behaviour but can have a destructive effect on both the individual and the group.

In a really difficult situation, it may be necessary to suspend the group and turn the session into a more formal talk. Sometimes using a task which will focus on the persistent problem may help the awkward person to get the problem 'off her chest'—her awkwardness may be her means of persisting until she gets the answer she wants.

SOME DOS AND DONT'S

DO
   — build on comment
   — find something to relate back to, a bridge back to the
      main area or a new direction
   — value each contribution
   — get the individual to be precise/specific or give an example

DON'T
   — be defensive when criticised
   — react emotionally
   — put people down — it is counterproductive
   — compete — trying to out-smart or win points
   — let it undermine confidence — it saps the positive
      energy

PERHAPS
   — if one or two people are dominating, split into smaller
      groups with specific tasks
   — if problems persist, suspend, task-explore, try to
      discuss whether there is a cause for the problems

OHT 31

Session Summary   This session has concentrated on the 'maintenance' aspect of groupwork by looking at some of the roles that people play in groups. It began with the suggestion that course members will have had experience of some people who they regard as being 'awkward', and continued by identifying some coping strategies — how to deal with them.

But the session went on to try to get their behaviour into perspective by asking how big the problem is and whose problem it is. The session ended by suggesting that it ought to be possible to see the individual in a positive light and turn her contribution to advantage in the discussion by maximising its potential. As teachers and group leaders refine their skills they will be better able to deal with group members who appear to hold different views, without feeling threatened.

Chapter Summary   Two areas have been covered in this chapter: (a) The need to keep up to date; the 'how' of this and its application to antenatal education. Other specialists can slot-in their own particular interests to this part of the course or, if the rest of the course is used as part of a training programme, these sessions could be omitted. (b) The evaluation of groupwork and strategies for maintaining group cohesion.

These sessions may help the course attenders to focus on the situations they will be dealing with when they go back to begin or continue their groupwork.

Resources

Balaskas J (1983) *Active Birth*. Unwin Paperbacks, London.

Balaskas J (1984) *The Active Birth Partner's Handbook*. Sidgwick & Jackson, London.

DeLyser F (1983). *Jane Fonda's Workout Book of Pregnancy, Birth and Recovery*. Allen Lane, London.

Dick-Read G (1966) *Antenatal Illustrated—the Natural Approach to Happy Motherhood*. Heinemann Medical Books, London.

Ebner M (1967) *Physiotherapy in Obstetrics*. Churchill Livingstone, Edinburgh.

Ebner M, McLaren J (1964) Teaching postnatal exercises. *Midwives Chronicle*, October, 1964. (Reprints available at 12p each + p&p) from: Midwives Chronicle, 98 Belsize Lane, London NW3 5BB.)

Family Doctor Publications. *Easier Childbirth—Psychoprophylaxis Method of Childbirth. Preparing Yourself for your Baby—Ante and Postnatal Exercises*. (BMA House, Tavistock Square, London WC1H 9JF.)

Heardman M (1982) *Relaxation and Exercise for Childbirth*. Revised by M Ebner. Churchill Livingstone, Edinburgh.

McKenna J, Polden M, Williams M (1980) *You—after Childbirth*. Churchill Livingstone, Edinburgh.

McLaren J (1975) *Preparation for Parenthood—Notes for Use with Antenatal Classes*. John Murray, London.

Obstetric Association of Chartered Physiotherapists Leaflets on ante and postnatal exercises.

Whiteford B, Polden M (1984) *Postnatal Exercises*. Century Publishing, London.

Williams M (1969) *Keeping Fit for Pregnancy and Labour*. (National Childbirth Trust, 9 Queenborough Terrace, London W2 3TB.)

Returning to the Community

7

This chapter focuses on the end of the course and the practitioners' return to the community or to teaching in hospital. The aim is to stimulate course participants into a consideration of how the course will affect their behaviour when they return to the field. The sessions are:
— theory into practice;
— teaching practice;
— 'Warm Fuzzies';
— the way ahead for the course;
— the way ahead for you.

The first session is didactic and needs to be relevant to the group attending the course, so the notes provided are brief. The example given for teaching practice is antenatal education, but it could be made relevant for any client/patient group. The course ends with two evaluation sessions preceded by the (optional) 'Warm Fuzzies' which is a short, lighthearted session.

Theory into Practice

AIM AND OBJECTIVE
AIM To provide attenders with information about continuing research in the district.
OBJECTIVE To identify local research which can be used when teaching in groups.

This session can include examples of externally-funded major research or minor individual projects carried out by student midwives, health visitors or other student groups. It can also involve health education or other projects undertaken by staff, such as tape/slide programmes or videotapes made to meet local needs. Both centres which have tried out the course have produced such material. In South Wales, one of the community midwives produced a tape/slide programme on *Information for Parents on the Obstetric and Midwifery Facilities available at Nevill Hall Hospital* (Nelmes 1983). A videotape on antenatal care has been made in Blackburn specifically for the Asian population.

Another example is that of a local project which was held on the use of videotapes in antenatal education, which included the theory behind the project and the practical working-out of a solution.

Relating this session to local needs, work and activities has been found to be useful and may possibly require its content to be changed as more up-to-date material becomes available.

Teaching Practice

AIM

To practise teaching antenatal mothers, using the skills learnt during the course, and to receive immediate feedback on performance.

OBJECTIVES

To allow course participants to practise their teaching skills and obtain feedback from their colleagues and the course leaders.

This session requires most of a morning to complete, and some time prior to the task for preparation.

Group task

Ideally, the groups will be small, with the midwife and health visitor who will be working together in the community presenting the session. Participants will have been told early in the course who they will be teaching with, and will be given or asked to choose a topic for the demonstration teaching session. The length of the session will depend on local factors such as the number of course attenders, the number of groups and the number of mothers who are willing to act as guinea pigs. Planning in advance will give time for the preparation of material, and access to visual aids within the precise time allocated for the session (practical details are discussed in Chapter 2).

For the actual teaching practice, some of the course members can act as observers in addition to the session presenters. Time should be allowed after the mothers have gone for feedback on teaching styles and techniques. One example of how feedback may be given is the playing back of a videotape of the session, a means of evaluation that is a very positive learning exercise for participants.

'Warm Fuzzies'

This is a pleasant session which may be omitted if there are time constraints.

AIM AND OBJECTIVE

AIM

To end the course on a positive note.

OBJECTIVE

To give the course members positive comments about themselves.

Group task

This task usually takes about 30 minutes and requires a clutter-free room to allow for easy movement. The leader distributes to each person a piece of Blutak and a sheet of paper large enough to allow everyone present to write something on it. All then stick the sheets of paper to each other's backs and write on those sheets one positive comment about each person, so that everyone will end up with a list of comments about herself written by her colleagues.

Feedback involves asking each participant to read to herself the comments written on her sheet. Whether or not the comments should then be read aloud depends on what the group decides; as the exercise is designed to promote positive rather than negative feelings some people may feel embarrassed by public disclosure. If this exercise precedes evaluation, it can provide a positive framework from which to begin.

The Way Ahead for the Course

AIM

AIM

To evaluate the course so that the different session leaders can gain immediate reactions to the course and receive suggestions for modifications which may be appropriate for subsequent courses.

This exercise may also provide a model of evaluation for the participants to use in their own classes. Methods of evaluation may vary. Each individual can be asked to comment on the course or small groups may work together to produce a composite evaluation. Headings may be provided such as 'most useful sessions', 'least useful sessions' and 'suggestions for improvement'.

The Way Ahead for You

AIM
AIM To translate the lessons learnt during the course into the practical reality of the world in which teaching will take place.

Local managers from both midwifery and health visiting (or other relevant groups) may be invited to this session to aid in the exchange of ideas and problems; the more managers who are present the wider will be the discussion. Participants are asked how they will apply the principles which have been discussed during the course and how they will effect change. Managers may be helped by knowing what their fieldworkers are trying to do, and why, and fieldworkers who may want to change the world overnight may come to appreciate the difficulties that managers have to contend with.

To effect change is notoriously difficult, its success hinging on the attitudes both of staff and of their managers. Immediately after a course, staff may be enthusiastic about introducing change both in the organisation and planning of teaching, and in the use of available facilities. The first can be difficult if other staff members who have not attended the course do not see the need for change. The second may be impossible if extra funding is required. Autocratic managers may determine what is taught and so negate the value of the course, especially if there is no opportunity for free discussion on both sides.

Summary   The sessions included here are those which bring the course to a close and have been found to be most effective as concluding sessions. They may assist three groups: firstly, the course leaders will discover if they have met the needs of the participants; secondly, the participants themselves will gain an opportunity to discuss the changes they would like to make. Thirdly, the presence of managers can be a stimulus to constructive discussion, especially if participants feel they have the support of other course members and leaders, and this can lead to better understanding between management and staff as each expresses a view on the need for change within managerial constraints.

Support for Course Leaders 8

The development of a course which makes extensive use of groupwork and experiential learning makes considerable demands on those who are organising and teaching/leading it. In addition, staff changes can cause problems. In Blackburn the course leader (the senior midwifery teacher) left to take up a new post once the first couple of courses had been put on. The new midwifery teacher experienced a feeling of panic as there was no-one to assist her with planning the next course in the series. Building support systems for the leaders will aid survival, and may enhance enthusiasm for innovation. A number of options are open for consideration.

Pool of Teachers

Where a number of teachers/leaders is available from the various professional groups (health education, nursing, health visiting and midwifery managers and teachers) the burden of running a course is not too heavy. Obviously this is easier for courses that are organised by a combination of health authorities. One method of ensuring continuity, used in South Wales, was to include several observers on each course who would take over as leaders of aspects of the next course. There are dangers here; firstly, if too many observers are in the room the atmosphere of the course may change so that group cohesiveness is affected, perhaps by the feeling of being under scrutiny. This can be avoided, in part, by asking the observers to become group members in all respects. More than two or three such members may cause an imbalance in the group, but in any event, the role of the observer must be clearly explained, i.e. that they, too, are with the group to learn but in a specific context. The second danger is that 'sitting next to Nellie' may not necessarily produce an effective teacher.

Training

If there is not enough expertise available with the Health Authority(ies) is it worth sending one or two members (perhaps from different professional groups) for training in specific skills—for instance coping with groups?

Documentation

Although this manual provides some documentation, its use as a resource can also be enhanced if the reasons for administrative and other decisions are recorded, perhaps by amplifying the checklist which follows. For instance, where two different venues have been tried, what were the advantages and disadvantages of each. Details such as the availability of car parking, or a sufficient number of electric sockets, may be the basis for a decision but if these are not recorded systematically they may, and probably will, be forgotten a few months, or years, later.

If the programme uses 'catchy' titles for sessions, for example, 'Shaping up to Motherhood' for the sessions designed to help midwives and health visitors to teach relaxation and exercises, record what these are and why so that a newcomer can see how they have been developed.

Checklist

* What is available in an individual authority?
* Is there sufficient expertise within the authority to start a course now?
* If not:
    — is it worth sending one member of health education or teaching staff on a course to help them to teach the field staff?
    — is this the point to consider pooling resources with another authority and putting on a joint course?
    — is there other expertise available locally — if necessary outside the NHS — for instance:
        — local NHS training support?
        — Further Education or Higher Education college?
        — voluntary organisations?
        (see also the resource lists)

Course
Evaluation

9

Pre-course Survey

Before the first training course was begun in Blackburn a consumer survey of 1000 mothers who delivered in a five-month period was undertaken; it was repeated after four courses had been held. The questionnaire used was an adapted version of that published by Perkins (1979b); it was distributed by the community midwives, who helped the mothers to complete it. The questionnaires were returned to the Nursing Officer, Community Midwifery, and computing of the responses was undertaken by the Health Authority. The results of the survey were used during the course as a basis on which to discuss local problems in antenatal education. One consequence of the survey was an increased appreciation of the needs of the Asian population—as previously mentioned, this led to the production locally of a videotape in response to these needs.

South Glamorgan had the advantage of a part-time research officer who was able to look at different aspects of their antenatal education service and copies of the reports of his work are still available (Rees 1981a&b; 1982). When considering change within the service, it might be worth trying to enlist the help of someone within the health authority who has had research experience.

Evaluating the Course

Course evaluation is essential if courses are to be improved, and a variety of methods can be used to achieve this end. Consideration should be given to the type of evaluation thought by course leaders to be the most pertinent; is the course designed to bring all the attenders up to a certain standard or will it encourage self-development so that skills improve according to individual capability?

Evaluation can be prepared for in advance, take place during the course or as a comprehensive exercise at the end.

Pre-course evaluation

Some of the evaluation can be begun during a pre-course meeting with participants, especially if it is organised on the 'What do you expect from this course?' lines. This may reveal those who are genuine volunteers, eager to attend, and those who resent being conscripted (if the latter are a regular feature, should not the course organisers discuss with managers why they are sending reluctant attenders?).

In-course evaluation

Evaluation is built into the course—for instance the sessions—'The way ahead for the course' or 'Where do we go from here?' on the last afternoon of the course invite verbal evaluation. The following are some of the questions that can be asked of the participants:

— what did you get out of this course, if anything?
— should the course be repeated?
— what improvements do you suggest?

More formal, written evaluation can involve the use of a number of different formats. For continuing evaluation during the course, two different formats (Forms 1 and 2) are shown below.

EVALUATION FORM 1

Please comment on the sessions held today

Session 1

Session 2

Session 3

Session 4

Session 5

EVALUATION FORM 2

Session title . . . .

DIRECTIONS

Please score your answers to the following questions on a scale of 1 to 7, 1 = low
and 7 = high, by encircling the appropriate numbers; for example, with question
1, if you found the ideas very interesting, you might circle 7, less interesting, a
lower number, down to 1 for not in the least interesting.

	Low						High
1 How interesting did you find the ideas in this session?	1	2	3	4	5	6	7
2 How practical or relevant were the suggestions made by the speakers?	1	2	3	4	5	6	7
3 To what extent do you feel you will make use of the information/ideas/suggestions?	1	2	3	4	5	6	7
4 Did you learn something in this session?	1	2	3	4	5	6	7

GROUPWORK ONLY

5 How productive was the groupwork	1	2	3	4	5	6	7
6 How productive was the reporting-back session?	1	2	3	4	5	6	7

Any useful comment: . . . .

The format presented in Form 2 has been used in South Wales throughout the courses
there. However, having to complete a questionnaire after each session of the day,
even when the time to do this is built into the schedule, adds considerably to the
load for the course members. This type of course, with its emphasis on experiential
learning and groupwork, can be very tiring for those who are unfamiliar with these
techniques, a factor that should be taken into consideration before using this method
of evaluation. Perkins (1981) asked her students for a report each day. Although her
initial experience was that the forms were completed and returned, these were
"dominated by such unilluminating comments as 'useful'."

Other problems of this type of evaluation are that forms are:
— unlikely to be returned regularly;
— may not be any use because course members are:
— exhausted
— apathetic
— actively hostile (Perkins 1981b).

In addition to this evaluation by participants, the teachers/leaders who are present
will be able to evaluate to a certain extent from their own perceptions. This is especially
true where there is team teaching so that the one not actively engaged in teaching
can note the reactions of the attenders, pick out the aspects which they do not
understand or dislike and gauge the 'feel' of the session. Observers—whether as
participants or not—can also be a useful means of feedback to those involved with

the teaching, although it must be remembered that no-one can observe everything and that views will, of necessity, be based on selective data.

Post-course evaluation

Examples of questionnaires used in post-course evaluation can be obtained from Rees (1982a—see resource list).

A post-course meeting where the attenders can express their feelings about the course can serve two purposes:

1 The course leaders can judge the useful aspects of the course, those which appealed to the attenders and those which they may have disliked but now realise were beneficial.
2 If managers are present the course attenders can discuss the practical applications of what they have learnt during the course to the 'real' world. Some of the difficulties they experience may point out the need for changes in the course. Alternatively, the course attenders may be able to discuss with their managers the reasons for their inability to make changes, obtain equipment, alter or adapt the facilities available.
3 There may be a need to 'debrief' the attenders to defuse any tension or aggravation which has arisen during the course or since it ended. The change from using familiar methods (such as a lecture) to involving the mothers in discussion and to ask questions, may leave the antenatal teachers with a feeling that their classes are less 'successful'. The skills learnt are not those which are acquired immediately during a week's course but have to develop over a period of time. The feeling of not being able to cope so well may mean that support is needed in the first few months.

Summary   Evaluation, either before starting a course or during it, needs to be considered in the light of local needs. Various means have been presented; development of the course to suit each participating health authority or group is dependent on the active evaluation and adaptation of the material presented here.

Development of Two Courses 10

The original development of a training manual in Nottingham was discussed in the introduction. There have been other initiatives in the past few years which mirrored the concern generated by the Leverhulme Health Education Project. A brief history of the developments in two different parts of the country demonstrates the activities undertaken to improve antenatal education services. Blackburn, Hyndburn and Ribble Valley Health Authority (since the 1982 reorganisation) approached the problem from the point of view of a single health authority whereas South Wales consisted of the combined efforts of four health authorities: South Glamorgan, Mid-Glamorgan, West Glamorgan and Gwent.

Developments in Blackburn

Blackburn, Hyndburn and Ribble Valley Health Authority serves a large population in heavily-industrialised as well as rural areas.

Following the NHS reorganisation in 1974 it became apparent to midwifery and health visiting managers that although parentcraft services were varied, they rarely met perceived needs of their clientele. As a result the Divisional Nursing Officers met to estimate the size of the task required to correct the situation and exchange ideas on possible solutions to the problems. The first stage in this initiative was concerned with:
—identifying problems;
—setting standards and guidelines; ·
—attempting to foster local working relationships.
The appointment of a Senior Health Education Officer (SHEO) in 1979 with experience in both midwifery and health visiting, provided a focus for this initiative. A critical appraisal of the services was encouraged, the new SHEO appreciating that little had improved despite the efforts since 1974. Midwifery and health visiting managers invited the SHEO to act as co-ordinator of an antenatal education working group.

Early meetings were exploratory, with the aim of exchanging ideas and cementing good personal relationships. The support of both the managers and the staff were needed since they would become involved in the subsequent implementation of proposed changes.

Awareness of the work of Perkins encouraged the working group to consider changes in their service, and at this stage the SHEO approached the Health Education Council (HEC) for assistance. Jane Randell of the HEC and Perkins of Nottingham agreed to join the working group to offer assistance.

There was, at this time, an awareness of the work in South Glamorgan, so it was suggested that the HEC should fund a research officer to work closely with Blackburn and South Glamorgan with the aim of undertaking a study of development in both areas. As a result, a research officer was appointed to the Department of Nursing, University of Manchester, under the direction of Ann Faulkner and Ann Thomson. Following this Blackburn stated that:

"The strategy of bringing in expertise from the Health Education Council and Manchester University Department of Nursing has given credibility to our efforts."

Blackburn outlined their priorities, which still hold in 1987 and are as follows:

(a) The need for a joint training programme for health visitors and midwives;
(b) The need to identify and examine the services provided;
(c) The need to turn the geographical problems to good effect by making use of flexible local approaches and applications of programmes;
(d) The need to foster mutual respect and acceptance between midwives and health visitors by educational means, and to influence good personal relationships on the sharing of parentcraft roles.
(e) to achieve common aims.

In addition to the ability to provide the resources, the means of achieving and evaluating these aims were still seen as a major task by those involved in the project.

The SHEO commented that she had been "able to observe change in personal relationships between professionals who work together and understand each other's roles in parentcraft education."

The prime requisites for those who seek to effect changes in the development of parentcraft education are, as in other fields, the qualities of:
— patience
— perseverance
— enthusiasm.

Developments in South East Wales

As part of the 'Year of the Child' in 1979, South Glamorgan Health Education Unit organised a day conference on 'Preparation for Parenthood' which was attended by a multidisciplinary group, who represented many aspects of antenatal experience. As a result of the conference the Health Authority was recommended to review the antenatal services in depth. A report is available (Rees 1979).

A survey was initiated by the Health Education Unit in South Glamorgan (Rees 1981a) of the three groups of midwives and health visitors involved in antenatal

education. This led to a series of recommendations for change which centred round three main areas:
- —the content and presentation of classes;
- —the timing and location of classes;
- —the publicity relating to classes.

Management gained an opportunity from these findings to identify priority areas within the structure of the hospital and community services.

It was recognised that publicity for the classes was poor so the working groups produced a series of posters, leaflets and invitation cards aimed at informing mothers-to-be and their partners about the facilities that were available. New classes were arranged in some areas, and the times of many existing ones altered, to meet the needs of the mothers. A significant change introduced by the working groups was to rename the classes *Ready-for-Baby Groups*.

The content and presentation of classes was recognised by the working groups to be in need of radical change and, as a result, they produced a series of recommendations for improvement. A major innovation was the recommendation by the groups that communication skills of midwives and health visitors should be improved. This led to the development of the antenatal education group-skills workshops. In addition:

"one of the reasons given by the professionals for the low numbers attending classes was the formal style of teaching. This was felt to deter many people from attending, particularly social classes four and five. In looking at possible areas for improvement, it was suggested that classes should be more informal, with women given greater encouragement to participate and discuss their needs and opinions". (Rees 1982)

To make the numbers on such a course viable without too much strain being placed on any one authority, a working party was set up consisting of Health Education Officers from South Glamorgan and West Glamorgan, who were later joined by those from Mid-Glamorgan and Gwent. Liaison with the HEC and Perkins led to agreement to test the training course devised by Perkins & Craig in South East Wales. The midwifery and health visiting managers agreed to send their staff on the course as well as to contribute to the teaching.

The series of courses held in each centre and attended both by midwives and health visitors led to the development of this manual. It has come from their practical experience, with contributions from those who taught and organised the courses. Both centres started from the basis of the course designed originally by Perkins & Craig (1981) but added to it or adapted it according to the needs of their own staff, and it is to be hoped that this manual will help others to do the same. Although there is more than enough material in it for any one course, tutors and organisers will be able to select what is relevant to the needs of their staff and the mothers, or other client groups that they seek to serve.

Appendix

Specimen Course Programmes

South Wales

DAY 1
1 Introduction to the course and each other
2 The views of midwives and health visitors
3 Creating an environment
4 "I never told them that"
5 Communication—dos and don'ts

DAY 2
1 Setting the scene—report by previous course members of changes made to their practice
2 Aims and objectives
3 Teaching and methods
4 Teaching a skill

DAY 3
1 Planning a session
2 How do groups work?
3 Triggers for discussion
4 Asking questions

DAY 4
1 Keeping up to date (i)—midwifery update
2 Keeping up to date (ii)

3 A mother's view: a session with invited postnatal mothers and their babies—some had attended antenatal classes and some had not
4 Importance of feedback

DAY 5
1 Awkward people
2 Theory into practice
3 The way ahead for you (session with the health visiting and midwifery managers—discussion about proposed changes on return to teaching)
4 The way ahead for the course (verbal evaluation of the course)

Blackburn

DAY 1
1 Individuals and groups
2 What preparations should be made?
3 Preparations (continued): the environment
4 What do we hope to achieve? (aims and objectives)
5 Evaluation of the day

DAY 2
1 Preparations: what teaching method should I use?
2 Getting it across—instructional techniques
3 Shaping up to motherhood (teaching relaxation and exercises)
4 Shaping up to motherhood (teaching relaxation and exercises)
5 Discussion regarding topics to be presented on the final day
6 Evaluation of the day

DAY 3
1 Everyone has something to say (groups)
2 Everyone has something to say (continued)
3 Interpretation of local research
4 Shaping up to motherhood (teaching relaxation and exercises)
5 Shaping up to motherhood (teaching relaxation and exercises—labour talk)
6 Evaluation of the day

DAY 4
1 Questions and answers
2 Listening and talking
3 Shaping up to motherhood (teaching relaxation and exercises)
4 Informal discussion of local issues
5 Shaping up to motherhood (teaching relaxation and exercises)
6 Did we get it right? (evaluation techniques)
7 Evaluation of the day.

DAY 5

1 Shaping up to motherhood (teaching relaxation and exercises—postnatal)
2 Parentcraft teaching—teaching practice with invited antenatal mothers
3 'Warm Fuzzies'—writing a good point about each member of the group on a piece of paper stuck on her back
4 Did we get it right and what do we do now? (session with the health visiting and midwifery managers—verbal evaluation of the course and discussion about proposed changes on return to teaching)

References and Resources

References

Those marked with ⋆ are the most useful references—those without are interesting background reading. For those references which have not been formally published, the source is given; prices (where shown) are those known to be correct at the time of going to press.

⋆Adams M E (1977) Providing a service. *Nursing Mirror Parentcraft supplement*, 29 Sept, 12-13.

Allen R (1981) *Pregnancy Groups—Alternatives to Antenatal Classes*. National Council for Voluntary Organisations.

⋆Anderson D C (ed) (1979) *Health Education in Practice*. Croom Helm, London.

Anderson D C , Fowler H K, Perkins E R & Spencer N J (1980) *Practical Prospects for Health Education in the 1980s*. Levehulme Health Education Project, University of Nottingham.

⋆Ashton R M & Crowe V J (1979) Development of programmes to prepare the midwife for education of parents for childbirth and parenthood. *Midwives Chronicle*, August, 248-250.

Bahl V (1984) Forging a new partnership. *Nursing Times*, 12 Sept, 19-20. (Linkworkers for antenatal care of Asians.)

Black P M, Faulkner A & Thomson A M (1984) Antenatal classes: a selective review of the literature. *Nurse Education Today*, 3(6) p, 130-133.

Black, P M, Booth K & Faulkner A (1984) Co-operation or conflict? How midwives and health visitors view each other's contribution to antenatal education. *Senior Nurse*, 1(33), 25-26.

⋆Boswell J (1979) Are classes 4 and 5 paying attention? *Nursing Mirror*, **148**(12), 24-25.

Boother D (1976) Antenatal defaulters. *Midwives Chronicle*, July, 170-171.

Boyd C & Sellars L (1982) *The British Way of Birth*, Pan Books, London.

Brammer A C (1977) Organised classes for pregnant women and their partners in preparation for childbirth and parenthood. *An Enquiry into the Classes Provided by the Maternity Services in England in 1975*. Maws Ed. Research Scholarship, 1974/75. (Available on loan from the RCM.)

Breese A C (1976) *Antenatal Classes and Preparation for Pregnancy, Birth and Motherhood.* M. Med. Sci dissertation, Nottingham University, (unpub.)

Brandenburger B (1976) Preparing for a happy birth. *Mother*, Aug, 40-41. (About the work of the NCT.)

Cartwright A (1979) *The Dignity of Labour.* Tavistock Publications, London.

Central Midwives Board (1962) *Handbook Incorporating the Rules of the CMB.*

Central Midwives Board (1980) *Handbook Incorporating the Rules of the CMB.*

*Chamberlain G (1975) Antenatal education: the consumer's view. *Midwife, Health Visitor and Community Nurse*, **11**(9), 289-92.

*Chamberlain G & Chave S (1977) Antenatal education. *Community Health*, **9**(1), 11-16.

*Clark J M & Stodulski A H (1978) How to find out: a guide to searching the nursing literature. *Nursing Times*, **74**(6), 21-23.

*Committee of Health and Social Security (1976) *Fit for the Future (Court Report).* HMSO, London.

Coyle A & Hicks C (1985) Elegance for pregnant mothers. *Nursing Mirror*, **159**(5), 1-4.

*Craven R D, Crouch M & Goosey R A (1975) Guidelines for teachers of parentcraft and relaxation (8 parts). *Midwives Chronicle*, Jan-Aug, 11-12; 55; 84-85; 118: 155; 205; 236; 266-267.

Davies I K (1973) *The Organisation of Training.* McGraw Hill, Maidenhead.

*Davies M (1977) Antenatal teaching. *Nursing Times*, 20 Oct, 1646-1647.

Department of Health and Social Security (1973) *The Family in Society, Preparation for Parenthood.* HMSO, London.

Draper J (1982) The level of preparedness for parenthood. *Maternal and Child Health*, **44**, 46-47.

*Draper J, Farmer S, Field S, Thomas H & Hare M J (1984) The working relationship between the health visitor and community midwife. *Health Visitor*, **57**; 366-368.

Ebner M (1967) *Physiotherapy in Obstetrics (including Education for Childbirth and Postnatal Restoration).* Churchill Livingstone, Edinburgh.

Elkind A K (1980) The nurse as health educator: the prevention and early detection of cancer. *Journal of Advanced Nursing*, **5**, 417-426.

*Ewles L & Simnett I (1985) *Promoting Health: A Practical Guide to Health Education.* John Wiley & Sons, Chichester.

Faulkner A (1980) *The Student Nurse's Role in Giving Information to Patients.* Unpublished M. Litt thesis, University of Aberdeen.

Faulkner A & Maguire P (1984) Teaching assessment skills. In Faulkner A (Ed) *Recent Advances in Nursing Communication.* Churchill Livingstone, Edinburgh.

Faulkner A & Maguire P (1986) *Assessment in the Community.* (In Press.)

Flanders N A (1970) *Analysing Teaching Behaviour.* Addison-Wesley Publishing Co, Reading, Massachusetts.

Gillett J (1976) A report on the survey on preparation for childbirth within the catchment area of Copthorne Maternity Unit, Shrewsbury. *International Journal of Nursing Studies*, **13**, 25-46.

Gillett J (1980) Teaching training through the National Childbirth trust. *Midwife, Health Visitor and Community Nurse*, 16 Sept, 380-381.

Hassid P (1984) *Textbook for Childbirth Educators.* Harper & Row, London.

Health Education Council (1982) *Major Programme for 1982-83.* Health Education Council, London.

Health Education Council (1984) *Major programme for 1984-85.* Health Education Council, London.

*Hyde B I (1982) Curriculum planning for antenatal health education. *Nurse Education Today*, **1**(6), 6-10.

Joint Board of Clinical Nursing Studies (1978) *Course Evaluation Package*. JBCNS, London.

Katona CLE (1981) Approaches to antenatal education. *Social Science in Medicine*, **15a**, 25-33.

Kerr M & McKee L 1981 The father role in child health care: is dad an expert, too? *Health Visitor*, **54**, 47-52.

Kirkham M J (1983) Labouring in the dark: limitations on the giving of information to enable patients to orientate themselves to the likely events and timescale of labour. In: Wilson-Barnett J. *Nursing Research: Ten Studies in Patient Care*. John Wiley & Sons, Chichester.

*Kitzinger S (1977) *Education and Counselling for Childbirth*. Bailliere Tindall, London.

Kuczynski H J (1984) Benefits of childbirth education—first stage of labour. *Midwives Chronicle*, **97**, 188-192. (American.)

Mager R F (1962) *Preparing Instructional Objectives*. Pitman Learning Inc, California.

*Macintyre S (1982) Communications between pregnant women and their medical and midwifery attendants. *Midwives Chronicle*, **95**, 387-395.

McLaren J (1975) *Preparation for Parenthood: Notes for Use with Antenatal Classes*. Murray, London.

Myles M (1985) *Textbook for Midwives*. Churchill Livingstone, Edinburgh.

National Association for Maternal and Child Welfare (NAMCW) (1977) *Parentcraft Teaching Aids*. (Information on literature, visual aids, professional associations, etc.)

National Childbirth Trust (undated) *Antenatal Teaching: Psychological Antenatal Preparation*. (Both single sheets available from NCT, 9 Queenborough Terrace, London W2 3TB.)

Nelmes V (1983) *Information for Parents on the Obstetric and Midwifery Facilities available at Nevill Hall Hospital*. Gwent Health Authority.

Nesbit J (1979) *Antenatal Language Kit to Teach English for Pregnancy*. Commission for Racial Equality.

*Nursing Mirror (1977) *Supplement on Parentcraft*. 29 Sept, 1-15.

Oakley A (1981) Adjustment to motherhood. *Nursing*, **1**, 899-901.

Oakley A & MacFarlane A (1980) A poor birthright. *New Society*, July, 172-173.

*Open University (1985) 1 *Leading a Group* (£4.50; a booklet, part of the Community Education Package). 2 *Family Life Styles* (£10.00; study pack). (Both available from: Learning Material Services Office (LMSO), Open University, PO Box 188, Walton Hall, Milton Keynes, MK7 6DH.)

Parents (1976) The ideal pregnancy (how knowledge and understanding can make childbirth easier). *Parents*, April, 8-12. (Available HEC 3536, old series.)

Perfrement S, (1984) New ideas for mothers and midwives. *Nursing Mirror Supplement*, 4 April, 1-3.

Parsons W D & Perkins E R (1982) Why don't women attend for antenatal care? *Midwives Chronicle*, October, 362-364.

Perkins E R (1977) *Community Nursing and Midwifery in the Sutton Area: Opportunities for Health Education*. Leverhulme Health Education Project Occasional Papers No. 5.

*Perkins E R (1978a) *Antenatal Classes in Nottinghamshire: the Pattern of Official Provision*. Leverhulme Health Education Project Occasional Papers No. 9.

*Perkins E R (1978b) *Having a Baby: an Educational Experience?* Leverhulme Health Education Project Occasional Papers No. 6.

*Perkins E R (1978c) *Group Health Education by Health Visitors*. Leverhulme Health Education Project Occasional Papers No. 7.

Perkins E R (1978d) *Networks and Dissemination: the Case for the Open University Parenthood Courses*. Leverhulme Health Education Project Occasional Papers No. 12.

Perkins E R (1978e) *Attendance at Antenatal Classes. A District Study*. Leverhulme Health Education Project Occasional Papers No. 13.

*Perkins E R (1979a) *What do Clients Need? Towards a Responsive Health Education Programme*. Leverhulme Health Education Project Occasional Papers No. 19.

The Leverhulme Health Education Project Occasional Papers and Nottingham Practical Papers in Health Education are available from: Nottinghamshire Health Education Unit, Huntingdon House, Huntingdon Street, Nottingham NG1 3LZ.

*Perkins E R (1979b) Monitoring antenatal classes: the development of a research tool. *Nursing Times*, 13 Dec, 2163-2169.

*Perkins E R (1979c) 'And did you go to classes, Mrs Brown?' *Midwives Chronicle*, **92**(1103), 422-425.

*Perkins E R (1979d) A look at the Open University parenthood courses. *Midwife, Health Visitor and Community Nurse*, June.

Perkins E R (1979e) *Parentcraft: a Comparative Study of Teaching Methods*. Leverhulme Health Education Project Occasional Papers No. 16.

*Perkins E R (1979f) Defining the need: an analysis of varying teaching goals in antenatal classes. *International Journal of Nursing Studies*, **16**, 275-282.

Perkins E R (1979g) *Teaching about Labour*. Leverhulme Health Education Project Occasional Papers No. 18.

Perkins E R (1980a) *Men on the Labour Ward*. Leverhulme Health Education Project Occasional Papers No. 22.

*Perkins E R (1980b) *Education for Childbirth and Parenthood*. Croom Helm, London.

*Perkins E R (1980c) The pattern of women's attendance at antenatal classes: is this good enough? *Health Education Journal*, **39**(1), 3-9.

Perkins E R (1980d) Preparation for childbirth: a role for physiotherapists in the community. *Association of Physiotherapists in Obstetrics and Gynaecology Newsletter*, Winter, 19-21.

Perkins E R (1981a) *The Individual Teacher: Learning to Improve*. Paper for limited circulation.

*Perkins E R (1981b) *Evaluating In-service Training: a Practical Approach*. Nottingham Practical Papers in Health Education, No. 3. University of Nottingham, Department of Adult Education/Nottinghamshire Health Education Unit.

*Perkins E R (1981c) Useful research—and the other kind (improving maternity services). *Health and Social Services Journal*, 23 January, 84-85.

Perkins E R (1982) *Developing Parentcraft Teaching*. Paper for limited circulation.

Perkins E R & Craig E (1981) *Parentcraft Teaching, the Basic Skills*. Paper for limited circulation.

Perkins E R & Morris B (1979) *Preparation for Parenthood: a Critique of the Concept*. Leverhulme Health Education Project Occasional Papers No. 17.

*Perkins E R & Morris B (1981) Should be prepare for parenthood? *Health Education Journal*, **40**(4) 107-110.

Pitcairn L (1978) Parents of the future. *Midwife, Health Visitor and Community Nurse*, **14**(11), 386-388.

*Prince J & Adams M E (1978) *Minds, Mothers and Midwives*. Churchill Livingstone, Edinburgh.

Prowse R (1981) A statistical survey of patient opinion concerning antenatal instruction. *Association of Chartered Physiotherapists in Obstetrics and Gynaecology. Newsletter No. 49*, Summer, 25-29.

Pugh G (1980) *Preparation for Parenthood—Some Current Initiatives*. National Children's Bureau, London.

Rathbone B (1973) *Focus on New Mothers: a Study of Antenatal Classes*. RCN, London.

*Rees C (ed) (1979) *Preparation for Parenthood: Report of a Day Conference*. South Glamorgan HA (T) Health Education Unit.

*Rees C (ed) (1981a) *A Review of Antenatal Education in South Glamorgan. The Findings of Three Working Groups*. South Glamorgan HA (T) Health Education Unit.

*Rees C (1981b) *Antenatal Services; the Views of Midwives and Health Visitors*. Proceedings of RCN Research Society XXII Annual Conference.

*Rees C (1982a) *"What did we Learn?" An Assessment of an Antenatal Education Group Skills Workshop*. South Glamorgan HA (T) Health Education Unit.
(Rees 1979, 1981a and 1982a are available from: Health Education Unit, St David's Hospital, Cowbridge Road East, Cardiff CF1 9TZ.)

*Rees C (1982b) Antenatal classes: time for a new approach. *Nursing Times*, **78**(34), 1446–1448.

*Rees C (1984) Asking questions. In: *Education and the Midwife Conference Report*. Association of Radical Midwives, London. (Available from ARM, 102 St Mary's Terrace, London W2 1SZ.)

Robinson S, Golden J & Bradley S (1983) *The Role and Responsibilities of the Midwife. NERU Report No. 1*. Chelsea College, University of London.

Roberts H, Wotten I D P, Kane K M & Harnett W E (1953) The value of antenatal preparation. *Journal of Obstetrics and Gynaecology of the British Empire*, **60**, 404–408.

Rodmell S & Smart (1982) *Pregnant at Work: the Experience of Women*. Open University/Kensington, Chelsea and Westminster Area Health Authority, 304 Westbourne Grove, London W1.

Rodway H E (1947) A statistical study on the effects of exercise for childbearing. *Journal of Obstetrics and Gynaecology of the British Empire*, **54**, 77–85.

Rogers J (1971) *Adults Learning*. Penguin Books, Middlesex.

Royal College of Midwives (1966) *Preparation for Parenthood*. RCM, London. (Available from Royal College of Midwives.)

Runswick H & Davis C C (1976) *Health Education: Practical Teaching Techniques*. Wiley HM + M Publishers, Chichester.

Russell G J (1973) *Teaching in Further Education*. Pitman Education Library, Pitman Publishing, London.

*Satow A & Evans M (1983) *Working with Groups*. Joint HEC/TACADE publication. (Available from TACADE, 2 Mount Street, Manchester M2 5NG.)

Smith J P (1979) The challenge of health education for nurses in the 1980s. *Journal of Advanced Nursing*, 5: 531–543.

Social Services Committee (1980) *Second Report on Perinatal and Neonatal Mortality (Short Report)*. HMSO, London.

Strehlow M S (1983) *Education for Health*. Harper & Row, London.

Sutherland I (1979) *Health Education: Perspectives and Choices*. George Allen & Unwin, London.

Tones BK (1978) *Effectiveness and Efficiency in Health Education: a Review of Theory and Practice*. Scottish Health Education Group Occasional Paper.

*Townsend P & Davidson N (1982) *Inequalities in Health (The Black Report)*. Pelican Books, Harmondsworth.

*Williams M & Booth D (1983) *Antenatal Education — Guidelines for Teachers*. Churchill Livingstone, Edinburgh.

Young C (1977) The need for parentcraft. *Nursing Mirror Supplement*, 29 Sept, 1–3.

Resources

Balaskas J (1983) *Active Birth*. Unwin Paperbacks, London.

Balaskas J (1984) *The Active Birth Partner's Handbook*. Sidgwick & Jackson, London.

Bountyvision (1987) Details of video programmes available, mainly suitable for use on postnatal wards. Available from Vinces Rd, Diss IP22 3HH.

DeLyser F (1983) *Jane Fonda's Workout Book of Pregnancy, Birth and Recovery*. Allen Lane, London.

Dick-Read G (1966) *Antenatal Illustrated—the Natural Approach to Happy Motherhood.* 3rd ed. Heinemann Medical Books, London.

Ebner M (1967) *Physiotherapy in Obstetrics.* 3rd ed Churchill Livingstone, Edinburgh.

Ebner M & McLaren J (1964) Teaching postnatal exercises. *Midwives Chronicle*, Oct. (Reprints available at 12p each (+p and p) from: Midwives Chronicle, 98 Belsize Lane, London NW3 5BB.)

Family Doctor Publications *Easier Childbirth—Psychoprophylaxis Method of Childbirth. Preparing Yourself for Your Baby—Ante and Postnatal Exercises.* (BMA House, Tavistock Square, London WC1H 9JF.)

Films, videos, and tape slide programmes are usually available from the local Health Education Unit or Department.

Gillet J (1985) A helping hand. *Senior Nurse*, **2**(5), 15–18. (A pull-out supplement listing support groups and organisations willing to provide pre and postnatal help and advice.)

Graves Medical Audiovisual Library: catalogue of tape and slide programmes. (Available from: Holly House, 220 New London Road, Chelmsford, Essex CM2 9BJ.)

Health Education Council trigger films—a set of 5 films each lasting about 10 minutes; aim to promote discussion concerning pregnancy, labour, pre and postnatal care, etc.

Heardman M (1982) *Relaxation and Exercise for Childbirth*, revised by M Ebner. Churchill Livingstone, Edinburgh.

Kohner N (1984) *Pregnancy*. Health Education Council, London. (A book with many pictures and diagrams about pregnancy, aimed at the first-time mother. Deals with the emotional side of childbirth, together with the physical aspects.)

McKenna J, Polden M & Williams M (1980) *You—after Childbirth*. A Churchill Livingstone Patient Handbook, Edinburgh.

McLaren J (1975) *Preparation for Parenthood—Notes for Use with Antenatal Classes.* John Murray, London.

Obstetric Association of Chartered Physiotherapists Leaflets on ante and postnatal exercises.

Parentcraft Education Teaching Aids. (Suggestions, sources, notes and guide for teachers. Available from: National Association for Maternal and Child Welfare, 1 South Audley Street, London W1Y 6JS.)

Various firms who promote baby products (such as Cow and Gate, Milton products, Farley's etc) produce a variety of tape slide programmes and films as well as flip charts.

Whiteford B & Polden M (1984) *Postnatal Exercises*. Century Publishing, London.

Williams M (1969) *Keeping fit for Pregnancy and Labour*. National Childbirth Trust, 9 Queenborough Terrace, London, W2 3TB.

Index

94